Management of Tardive Dyskinesia

Collected Articles from H&CP

Contents

Foreword

The identification, effective management, and ultimate prevention of tardive dyskinesia demand that clinicians be up to date on issues related to this serious movement disorder. Yet the large body of literature on tardive dyskinesia contains relatively few articles designed to meet clinicians' needs for timely, practical information on diagnosis and management. This collection of articles, published by the Hospital and Community Psychiatry Service, contains information on tardive dyskinesia that we believe helps meet these needs of clinicians. All the articles originally appeared in *Hospital and Community Psychiatry*.

The first article, an overview of tardive dyskinesia, covers such important issues as definition and differential diagnosis, factors that predispose patients taking neuroleptics to the disorder, suspected etiologic mechanisms, and patient management. The overview is followed by a review of studies of the use of intermittent therapy in tardive dyskinesia and then by a discussion of tardive dyskinesia within the broader context of movement disorders.

Other articles consider the sources of resistance to talking with patients about tardive dyskinesia, discuss the increasing legal risks of failing to take proper precautions in administering neuroleptics and to obtain informed consent, describe how to differentiate between subtypes of tardive dyskinesia and between tardive dyskinesia and other movement disorders, and present guidelines for the physical management of patients with certain symptoms. Finally, there is a brief statement by APA's Task Force on Tardive Dyskinesia summarizing information about the disorder and containing recommendations for the use of neuroleptics.

We believe that, taken together, these articles reflect the current state of knowledge and practice concerning tardive dyskinesia. We hope you find them helpful.—H. RICHARD LAMB, M.D.

Dr. Lamb is professor of psychiatry at the University of Southern California School of Medicine at Los Angeles and chairman of the Committee to Coordinate the H&CP Service, Journal, and Institute.

An Update on Tardive Dyskinesia

George M. Simpson, M.D.
Edmond H. Pi, M.D.
John J. Sramek, Pharm.D.

The authors review recent research on definition, diagnosis, neuropathophysiology, treatment, management, and factors that increase risk of tardive dyskinesia, a severe and often unremitting movement disorder associated with neuroleptic treatment. Supersensitivity of dopamine receptors is believed to be the cause of tardive dyskinesia, and treatment strategies have consisted of pharmacologic blockade of dopamine receptors, depletion of dopamine, and restoration of the balance between the dopaminergic system and the neurotransmitter systems that regulate it. Several experimental neuroleptics that do not appear to cause tardive dyskinesia may be approved for use in the United States, but for now preventive measures, such as wise prescription and gradual tapering of neuroleptics, as well as careful monitoring for symptoms of tardive dyskinesia are the clinician's best defense.

Dr. Simpson is professor and director of clinical psychopharmacology in the department of psychiatry of the Medical College of Pennsylvania, 3200 Henry Avenue, Philadelphia, Pennsylvania 19129. Dr. Pi is associate professor of psychiatry and director of adult psychiatry at the University of Southern California School of Medicine. Dr. Sramek is drug information specialist and director of pharmaceutical services at Metropolitan State Hospital in Norwalk, California.

The introduction of neuroleptic agents in the early 1950s ushered in a period of therapeutic optimism. It had a profound effect on psychiatric practice and stimulated much biomedical research (1,2). Soon after, abnormal movements, later named tardive dyskinesia, were observed in patients taking neuroleptics (3,4).

Although identification of tardive dyskinesia came early, widespread recognition and concern among clinicians followed more slowly. Today tardive dyskinesia is the subject of much research and is widely recognized as the major side effect of neuroleptics.

This article discusses the currently unresolved issues of the tardive dyskinesia syndrome, with emphasis placed on clinical management. A survey of the literature on neuropathophysiology and its implications for treatment is presented.

Definition of tardive dyskinesia

Research has played a large and as yet unfinished role in changing our concept of tardive dyskinesia. Recent research has focused on providing a more critical definition of the syndrome. Originally abnormal movements of the face, mouth, and tongue, the so-called buccolingual masticatory syndrome, were considered the defining symptoms of tardive dyskinesia. Now choreathetoid movements of the hands, feet, and arms and respiratory dyskinesia are accepted as part of the syndrome (5).

A variety of standardized measuring devices developed for use in prospective studies, clinical trials, and epidemiological surveys represent a real advance in the evaluation and understanding of tardive dyskinesia (6,7). Much effort has gone into distinguishing withdrawal tardive dyskinesia from persistent tardive dyskinesia (8,9). From the earliest use of neuroleptics it has been known that tardive dyskinesia often appears after a neuroleptic has been withdrawn and that in many of these cases the condition improves or disappears (10–12). The rate of disappearance of withdrawal tardive dyskinesia has been quoted as being anywhere from 0 to 90 percent (13). This wide disparity suggests that different populations were studied or, at the very least, different methodologies were used.

Suffice it to say that if we were to abruptly withdraw neuroleptics from a large number of subjects, a large percentage would develop a dyskinesia, particularly if they had been on high dosages. In a substantial number of those subjects, the dyskinesia would disappear in weeks, in months at most. Persistent tardive dyskinesia occurs when dyskinetic movements persist for more than three months after withdrawal of neuroleptics. Research diagnostic criteria have been developed to clarify withdrawal and persistent tardive dyskinesia (14).

Differential diagnosis

Much information about the differential diagnosis of tardive dyskinesia has accrued, but a simple pathological sign for tardive dyskinesia has yet to be identified. There is new evidence that oral dyskinesia, a common symptom of tardive dyskinesia, may occur in drug-free elderly populations at a rate higher than the early estimate of 2 percent (15). One study estimated the incidence of oral dyskinesia in a nursing home population never treated with neuroleptics to be as high as 37 percent (16). This finding suggests that the oral symptoms of elderly patients on neuroleptics may not always be due to tardive dyskinesia.

At the same time, there are reports that nonneuroleptic drugs, including antihistamines, phenytoin, and tricyclic antidepressants, are on rare occasions associated with tardive dyskinesia (17–19).

Other disorders, such as stereotyped movement of schizophrenia, Gilles de la Tourette's syndrome, Wilson's disease, atypical torsion dystonias, and Huntington's chorea, can be confused with tardive dyskinesia (5). Distinguishing tardive dyskinesia from some of these progressively degenerative conditions is its stability over time. After the onset of tardive dyskinesia, there is a reasonably long period during which symptoms do not change. Indeed, studies have shown that even with continued neuroleptic use, tardive dyskinesia may decrease over time. Assessment of the patient's history and the characteristic features and progression of the condition could help the clinician make a differential diagnosis.

Rabbit syndrome, a rare condition characterized by rapid tremor of the lips, was initially included as a symptom of tardive dyskinesia, then excluded when it was shown to respond to antiparkinson agents (20). However, it is still considered a side effect of long-term neuroleptic use, but one that is always reversible.

Another syndrome that may be confused with tardive dyskinesia is tardive dystonia, a very rare disorder that affects young adults after only brief exposure to neuroleptics. It tends to affect the neck muscles first, and its presenting symptoms are usually opisthotonus or abnormal head position. To that extent it is similar to the acute dystonic reactions that patients may develop early in neuroleptic treatment. However, tardive dystonia is a persistent condition that usually does not disappear when neuroleptics are withdrawn.

We have observed that abnormal tongue movements are absent early in the course of tardive dystonia, but they can develop later in a small number of cases, perhaps in association with high doses of anticholinergics that are used to treat the condition. The spasm of the neck muscles in tardive dystonia is prolonged and may extend to muscles of the shoulder girdle and, ultimately, of the trunk. In extreme cases, the subject's head may be continuously retracted so that walking is virtually impossible and on direct frontal view the subject's face and eyes are not visible. Such patients rest their heads against solid objects in an attempt to relieve the spasms and may walk in close contact with a wall. Movements may interfere with the patient's eating. Hemiballistic arm movements may occur, but the patient may be able to modify them so that they appear purposeful.

There is no definitive treatment for tardive dystonia. High doses of anticholinergics are claimed to be of benefit (21), but we have found most patients do not respond to them. Trials of baclofen and high doses of benzodiazepines, such as clonazepam, have been attempted with varying degrees of success. If dystonias are extreme and severe, restarting of neuroleptics may be required. Some cases of tardive dystonia may represent late-onset congenital torsion dystonias that were provoked or unmasked by neuroleptics. In those cases treatment would be the same as for torsion dystonias.

Predisposing factors

Increasing age is the most consistent risk factor for tardive dyskinesia (22,23). This finding has yet to be explained but may be related to pathological changes in the brain associated with the aging process, which have also been demonstrated in animals (24).

There is a higher prevalence of tardive dyskinesia among women, mainly in upper age groups. The reason for this difference is unclear (25). It has been postulated that estrogen, which modulates dopamine receptor sensitivity, may protect younger women from tardive dyskinesia (26,27).

Except for age and sex, factors that increase vulnerability to tardive dyskinesia remain uncertain (28–31). However, the reports of tardive dyskinesia in young adults following brief exposure to neuroleptics (10) and of early onset of severely debilitating tardive dyskinesia in children and adolescents taking neuroleptics (32) indicate that individual susceptibility must play a large role in the development of tardive dyskinesia.

Several studies have suggested that higher doses of neuroleptics may be related to higher prevalence and severity of tardive dyskinesia (29,33–35). Other studies, including a transcultural study, have not confirmed that correlation (28,31,36). Recently a low prevalence and a lack of severe forms of tardive dyskinesia in patients who were treated with very low doses of depot fluphenazine were reported (37). It has been suggested that neuroleptic drug holidays may increase the risk of developing tardive dyskinesia (38,39).

Virtually all available neuroleptics have been associated with tardive dyskinesia. Efforts to identify classes of neuroleptics that pose a higher risk have produced inconclusive and confusing results (38–41). For instance, some authors have claimed depot forms of neuroleptics, such as fluphenazine decanoate, increase the risk of tardive dyskinesia (42,43), but other authors have claimed depot forms are associated with a lower risk of tardive dyskinesia than oral neuroleptics (44). Low-potency neuroleptics have also been reported to pose a greater risk for tardive dyskinesia (45). All of these data must be interpreted cautiously; none represent convincing evidence that any one neuroleptic is more or less likely to be associated with tardive dyskinesia.

One study found higher plasma levels of neuroleptics in patients with tardive dyskinesia compared with those without tardive dyskinesia (46), suggesting that tardive dyskinesia patients do not metabolize neuroleptics as efficiently as patients who do not develop tardive dyskinesia. Again, contradictory data were reported by other investigators (47).

The relationship of tardive dyskinesia to another side effect of neuroleptic drugs, parkinsonism, and of the drugs used to treat it has been carefully evaluated (48,49). Several studies have described the coexistence of tardive dyskinesia and parkinsonism (50–52). Recent data have lent renewed support to an early idea that the severity of a patient's parkinsonism could predict whether the patient would develop tardive dyskinesia (37), a concept that studies over the years have failed to confirm (40,53–55). Contrary to speculation, antiparkinson agents have not been shown to predispose patients to tardive dyskinesia, although they may exacerbate or unmask it (56).

It has also been claimed that patients suffering from affective disorders are at greater risk for developing tardive dyskinesia than are patients who have other psychiatric disorders.

One recent study reported a high prevalence of spontaneous voluntary movement disorders in elderly nursing home patients who had never been treated with neuroleptics (16). Another study found no difference in the incidence of tardive dyskinesia among chronic schizophrenics who had never received neuroleptics and those who had received them (57). A difference was found between the two groups when data were

corrected for age, but it clearly was not as striking as one might expect. The study suggests that chronic schizophrenia itself may predispose one to tardive dyskinesia.

Neuropathophysiology and treatment implications

Although the exact etiologic mechanism behind tardive dyskinesia remains unknown (58), the most accepted theory involves supersensitivity of dopamine receptors in the basal ganglia following prolonged neuroleptic administration (59). Supersensitivity of dopamine receptors in the limbic system may also be related to the neuropathological changes that often accompany tardive dyskinesia, but much more research is needed to verify that hypothesis. Certainly the existence of withdrawal dyskinesia after discontinuation of neuroleptic drugs argues in favor of the dopamine receptor supersensitivity theory. Much of the evidence for this theory comes from pharmacological studies employing agonists and antagonists of the various neurotransmitter systems.

Dopaminergic system. Pharmacological studies of the dopaminergic system indicate that dopamine agonists worsen tardive dyskinesia while dopamine antagonists, or dopamine blockers, improve it, if only temporarily. Numerous double-blind studies have shown that dopamine antagonists are initially effective in ameliorating the symptoms of tardive dyskinesia (60,61), but often their use results eventually in further worsening of symptoms, so that their clinical usefulness is severely limited. Nevertheless, these drugs may be helpful in selected cases, such as that of an elderly patient with incapacitating tardive dyskinesia.

There has been much interest of late in the newer dopamine antagonists, including clozapine, pimozide, oxiperomide, and sulpiride, antipsychotic agents that may act selectively at dopamine receptor sites not linked to adenylate cyclase (62). The effectiveness of some of these antischizophrenic

agents in reducing tardive dyskinesia symptoms without significantly aggravating parkinsonism argues for the existence of two separate populations of dopamine receptors involved in the control of extrapyramidal function (63,64), which has been demonstrated in an animal model (65).

Clozapine is currently being considered for introduction in the U.S. However, the possibility exists that clozapine may also induce tardive dyskinesia (66); careful long-term study of that possibility will be required even if the drug is approved and the risk of agranulocytosis accompanying its use is deemed acceptable. The possibility of using lithium in combination with neuroleptics to prevent tardive dyskinesia is also exciting (67), and we eagerly await further reports. However, controlled studies indicate that lithium is not as effective a treatment for tardive dyskinesia as was first thought, even when treatment continues for one year (68,69).

Another treatment for tardive dyskinesia involving the dopaminergic system consists of altering the presynaptic transmission of dopamine using dopamine-depleting drugs, such as reserpine. Although not available in the U.S., one such drug, tetrabenazine, has been successful in several controlled studies (70,71). Tetrabenazine appears to have more selective effects on central nervous system activity and has fewer hypotensive effects than reserpine, but its use may be limited by a decline in patients' rate of improvement with long-term administration (72). Dopamine-depleting drugs may be most successful in improving severe symptoms (21), but they can also exacerbate underlying psychiatric illness (73) and, in presumably rare cases, even cause tardive dyskinesia.

There have been conflicting reports about the use of L-dopa, a dopamine agonist, to treat tardive dyskinesia. Although one study indicated moderate improvement with higher dosages, the improvement was canceled out by simultaneous administration of dopamine antagonists, such as neuroleptics, needed for control of psychotic symptoms (74).

Biochemical changes in tardive dyskinesia have been reported. Plasma levels of monoamine oxidase levels were reportedly lower and plasma levels of dopamine beta-hydroxylase were reportedly higher in patients with tardive dyskinesia than in those without tardive dyskinesia (75,76). It has also been reported that the addition of disulfiram, which stimulates release of dopamine beta-hydroxylase, was associated with improvement in tardive dyskinesia (39).

Cholinergic system. If the dopaminergic system plays a role in the development of tardive dyskinesia, then acetylcholine can be seen as a modulator of the expression of the disorder because acetylcholine inhibits dopamine. Therefore, restoring the balance between dopamine and acetylcholine with cholinergic drugs should improve tardive dyskinesia. Indeed, physostigmine, an anticholinesterase, has been shown to improve tardive dyskinesia (77), but because physostigmine requires intravenous administration and is effective for only a short time, the finding is of little clinical value. Tacrine, an orally active anticholinesterase, has been shown to reduce tardive dyskinesia significantly more than placebo in a short-term study (78).

Oral cholinergics have been tried in tardive dyskinesia, but their use must still be considered experimental. Conflicting reports of the effectiveness of deanol, one of the first oral cholinergics used, are best viewed with the present knowledge that deanol's activity and mode of action are much in question. Lecithin (phosphatidyl choline), which has fewer side effects than choline, has subsequently been studied as a possible treatment for tardive dyskinesia, but it remains unclear whether lecithin is cholinomimetic. In one recent controlled double-blind study of choline in 11 patients with persistent tardive dyskinesia, seven showed partial or minimal improvement, two did not change, and two worsened (79). Positive results were obtained in two other controlled studies (80,81). Lecithin has been reported to be effective in several uncontrolled studies (82,83).

The possibility of using lithium in combination with neuroleptics to prevent tardive dyskinesia is also exciting, and we eagerly await further reports.

The role of acetylcholine in tardive dyskinesia was first suggested by the observation that anticholinergics fail to improve tardive dyskinesia and, indeed, usually worsen or precipitate it. Administration of anticholinergic drugs to patients taking neuroleptics has been proposed as a strategy for early detection of tardive dyskinesia (52). Intravenous administration of the anticholinergic benztropine, however, had no significant effect in one controlled double-blind study, although oral benztropine did increase dyskinetic movements (84). Clinically an exacerbation of abnormal movements is often seen when anticholinergics are used in tardive dyskinesia, but a recent review of the literature does not support the earlier claim that these drugs are a risk factor in the development of tardive dyskinesia (56).

GABAergic system. Agonists of gamma-aminobutyric acid (GABA), a neurotransmitter that like acetylcholine is an inhibitor of dopamine transmission, have also been advocated in the treatment of tardive dyskinesia. The lack of clear results of studies of GABA agonists may be attributable to the uncertain or mixed mechanisms of actions of these drugs. The benzodiazepines appear to facilitate GABA transmission, but there have been conflicting reports of their success in treating tardive dyskinesia (85,86). We have often used diazepam in studies of neuroleptics and tardive dyskinesia in the drug-withdrawal period, but we have found it to have no effect in reducing the severity of tardive dyskinesia (41).

Baclofen, which may act directly on GABA, has also produced mixed results. One study claimed that baclofen may be helpful for patients with truncal tardive dyskinesia but that the appearance of unwanted side effects usually warrants its discontinuation (87). The results of trials of valproic acid in tardive dyskinesia are also conflicting; doses as high as 2100 mg per day may be needed to produce an effect (88). Enthusiasm was initially expressed about muscimol, a GABA agonist, and further results are anxiously awaited. However, there are reports that muscimol exacerbates psychosis (89). More recently analogues of GABA, including gamma-acetylenic GABA and gamma-vinyl GABA, have been shown to be moderately effective in tardive dyskinesia (66,90).

Other neurotransmitter systems. In general, controlled studies of a large number of other drugs for tardive dyskinesia have failed to substantiate early claims of success. Recently improvement in tardive dyskinesia has been reported with clonidine alone and in combination with bromocriptine, which may indicate that the noradrenergic system has a role in the pathophysiology of tardive dyskinesia (91,92). There have also been claims for the effectiveness of L-tryptophan and other serotonergic agents, but very little data are available to implicate the serotonergic system in tardive dyskinesia.

Management of tardive dyskinesia

The previous discussion should have made it apparent that there is no single satisfactory treatment for tardive dyskinesia. Claims of effec-

Figure 1
Scheme for clinical management of tardive dyskinesia

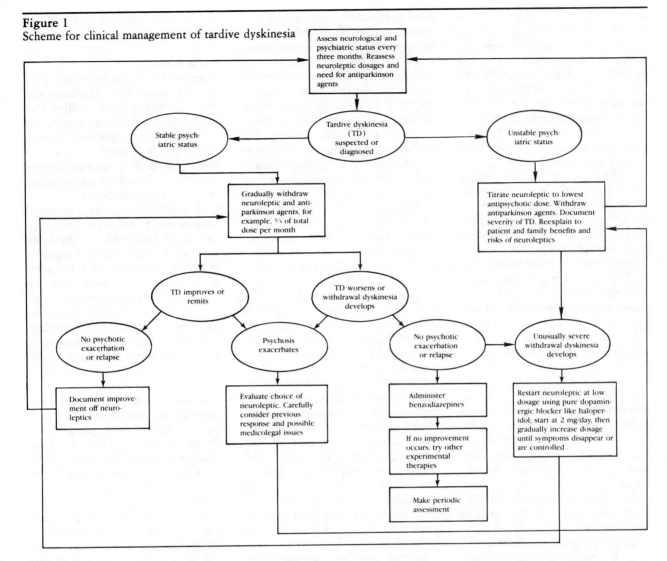

tive treatment are inconsistent and vary widely, perhaps owing to the fact that even if certain treatments are statistically effective, their clinical effect is often small. One has to be optimistic about the possible availability in the U.S. of neuroleptics such as clozapine that may not produce tardive dyskinesia. At present, however, we can only use existing drugs wisely, for treatment of disorders in which they are of proven benefit and superior to alternative strategies—schizophrenia, acute mania, and perhaps organic disorders. Figure 1 diagrams clinical management of tardive dyskinesia.

Whenever neuroleptics are employed, it is important to prescribe the lowest effective dosage and look for early signs of tardive dyskinesia. The best preventive measure is early detection, and a number of brief rating scales (6,7) may be used periodically to assess neurological status.

Clinicians should watch for changes in facial movements, checking periodically for abnormal movements of the tongue within the buccal cavity. Tongue movements are best detected by asking the patient to stand with mouth open and eyes closed and to tap his thumbs against each of his fingers. There are no pathognomonic signs for tardive dyskinesia, but abnormal tongue movements are considered to be the best early indicator. If depot fluphenazine is being given, it is best to test for tardive dyskinesia at a standard time relative to the injection schedule.

In the past routine drug holidays were advocated as a means of unmasking and even preventing tardive dyskinesia. They are no longer recommended, as several studies have correlated drug-free intervals with increased risk of tardive dyskinesia (38,39,93,94). Those findings, however, should not discourage clinicians from initiating a trial period of drug withdrawal in the hope of discontinuing the drug altogether.

Even if one is careful in using neuroleptics and makes frequent preventive assessments, a certain percentage of patients taking neuroleptics will develop tardive dyskinesia. When faced with the suspicion or diagnosis of tardive dyskinesia, the most logical course is to discontinue the neuroleptic. However, that may not be possible or desirable in patients for whom there is no effective treatment alternative and to whom psychiatric illness poses greater harm than does tardive dyskinesia. Numerous nonneuroleptic treatments of schizophrenia, such as propranolol, clonidine, lithium, and calcium channel blockers, have been advocated, but at present these therapies must be considered experimental. The clinician must carefully assess each case and consider all information about the patient, including the severity of the psychiatric illness, the number of hospitalizations, and the availability and need for social support systems.

In most cases the patient's psychiatric status will determine the management of tardive dyskinesia. If the psychiatric status is not stable—for instance, if the patient is psychotic—continued prescribing of neuroleptics may be necessary. However, one can minimize the risk of further development of tardive dyskinesia by reducing the dosage to the lowest effective amount and withdrawing antiparkinson agents slowly over two to three weeks.

Continuation of the neuroleptic must be repeatedly assessed and documented. Consideration should be given to alternative treatments for the psychosis, both drug and nondrug. Curiously, tardive dyskinesia can improve even when the patient is receiving continuous neuroleptic treatment, but there is no way of predicting whether a patient will improve, remain unchanged, or worsen. Patients who have simultaneous tardive dyskinesia and idiopathic Parkinson's syndrome present a disconcerting dilemma to the clinician, who must often discontinue all medications to determine which condition is more disabling.

If the patient's psychiatric status is stable, neuroleptics can be discontinued by reducing the dosage gradually, by approximately one-third per month. Even moderately severe tardive dyskinesia can disappear completely after withdrawal of neuroleptics. However, remission of abnormal movements is unpredictable and often requires patience. In a recent drug-discontinuation study of schizophrenic and nonschizophrenic patients, the probability of achieving a 50 percent reduction in a patient's abnormal movements was estimated to be 87 percent if the patient could be kept off neuroleptics for at least 18 months (95). Antiparkinson agents, seldom required in chronic patients, should also be withdrawn slowly over two to three weeks. Abrupt withdrawal may cause withdrawal symptoms (96).

During the drug-withdrawal phase tardive dyskinesia may worsen, and it may be necessary to slow the withdrawal and/or add a benzodiazepine, such as diazepam (15 to 30 mg per day), to temporarily ease the muscular discomfort of tardive dyskinesia and allay the patient's anxiety about worsening of the dystonic movements. If the psychosis also worsens at this time or the tardive dyskinesia is unusually severe, neuroleptic dosage may have to be increased. If the neuroleptic has already been completely withdrawn, it may have to be restarted.

In such instances, we prefer to use a high-potency drug like haloperidol, based on our experience that potent dopamine-blocking drugs with less anticholinergic activity are easier to titrate. Low-potency neuroleptic drugs, such as chlorpromazine or thioridazine, are more difficult to withdraw in chronic patients. Their withdrawal often leads to other complaints, such as insomnia and anxiety (97).

If tardive dyskinesia becomes worse but is not severely incapacitating following withdrawal of neuroleptics, and there is no exacerbation or relapse of psychosis, the use of benzodiazepines or other experimental therapies are preferred to the reintroduction of neuroleptics. The more benign and promising treatments, such as the GABAergic agonists and lecithin, should be attempted first.

Conclusions

Tardive dyskinesia remains a perplexing problem for clinicians and for patients and their families. Despite considerable research, no new risk factors have been identified. Elderly females are most at risk, and there is some evidence that higher dosages of neuroleptics may also be a risk factor.

A multitude of experimental treatments have been evaluated but none has been a convincing success. Recent evidence suggests that the outcome of long-term neuroleptic treatment may be more benign than previously supposed if great care is taken to monitor the amount of neuroleptics administered. Studies have shown patients with tardive dyskinesia who continued to receive neuroleptics in the least amount necessary to control psychosis in general did not worsen. In fact many improved over an eight-year follow-up period. Until we have other treatments for schizophrenia or antipsychotic agents that do not produce tardive dyskinesia, the emphasis must be on prevention.

All neuroleptics appear equally likely to suppress the symptoms of schizophrenia and to cause tardive dyskinesia. Therefore care should be taken to prescribe neuroleptics only to patients for whom no other treatment is effective. Clinicians should attempt to reduce the dosage required to treat acute episodes early in treatment. They should carefully monitor for signs of tardive dyskinesia and attempt to reduce or even withdraw the neuroleptics.

References

1. Romano J: Psychiatry and medicine. Annals of Internal Medicine 79:582–588, 1960
2. Snyder SH: Basic science of psychopharmacology, in Comprehensive Textbook of Psychiatry, 3rd ed. Edited by Kaplan HI, Freedman AM, Sadock BJ. Baltimore, Williams & Wilkins, 1980
3. Sigwald J, Bouttier D, Raymond C, et

al: Quatre cas de dyskinesie, facio-bucco-linguo-masticatrice a l'evolution prolongee secondaire a un traitement par les neuroleptiques. Revue Neurologie (Paris) 100:751–755, 1959

4. Uhrbrand L, Faurbye A: Reversible and irreversible dyskinesia after treatment with perphenazine; chlorpromazine; reserpine; ECT therapy. Psychopharmacologia 1:408–418, 1960

5. Simpson GM, Pi EH, Sramek JJ: Adverse effects of antipsychotic agents. Drugs 21:138–151, 1981

6. Simpson GM, Lee JH, Zoubok B, et al: A rating scale for tardive dyskinesia. Psychopharmacology 64:171–179, 1979

7. Early Clinical Drug Evaluation Unit, National Institute of Mental Health: Abnormal Involuntary Movement Scale (AIMS). Intercom 4:3–6, 1975

8. Kazamatsuri H, Chien C-P, Cole JO: Treatment of tardive dyskinesia, II: short-term efficacy of dopamine-blocking agents haloperidol and thiopropazate. Archives of General Psychiatry 27:100–103, 1972

9. Kennedy PF, Herson HL, McGuire RJ: Extrapyramidal disorders after prolonged phenothiazine therapy. British Journal of Psychiatry 118:509–518, 1971

10. Simpson GM: Tardive dyskinesia (ltr). British Journal of Psychiatry 122:618, 1973

11. Crane GE: Rapid reversal of tardive dyskinesia (ltr). American Journal of Psychiatry 130:1159, 1973

12. Moline RA: Atypical tardive dyskinesia. American Journal of Psychiatry 132:534–535, 1975

13. American College of Neuropsychopharmacology—Food and Drug Administration Task Force: Neurological syndromes associated with antipsychotic drug use (edtl). Archives of General Psychiatry 28:463–466, 1973

14. Schooler NR, Kane JM: Research diagnoses for tardive dyskinesia. Archives of General Psychiatry 39:486–487, 1982

15. Varga E, Sugerman AA, Varga V, et al: Prevalence of spontaneous oral dyskinesia in the elderly. American Journal of Psychiatry 139:329–331, 1982

16. Delwaide PJ, Desseilles M: Spontaneous buccolinguofacial dyskinesia in the elderly. Acta Neurologica Scandinavica 56:256–262, 1977

17. Davis WA: Dyskinesia associated with chronic antihistamine use (ltr). New England Journal of Medicine 294:113, 1976

18. Chadwick D, Reynolds EH, Marsden CD: Anticonvulsant-induced dyskinesia: a comparison with dyskinesias induced by neuroleptics. Journal of Neurology 39:1210–1218, 1976

19. Fann W, Sullivan JL, Richman B: Dyskinesias associated with tricyclic antidepressants. British Journal of Psychiatry 128:490–493, 1976

20. Jus K, Jus A, Gautier J, et al: Studies of the actions of certain pharmacological agents on tardive dyskinesia and on the rabbit syndrome. International Journal of Clinical Pharmacology 9:138–145, 1974

21. Fahn S: Treatment of tardive dyskinesia: use of dopamine-depleting agents. Clinical Neuropharmacology 6:151–158, 1983

22. Smith JM, Kucharski LT, Eblen C, et al: An assessment of tardive dyskinesia in schizophrenic outpatients. Psychopharmacology 64:99–104, 1979

23. Smith JM, Baldessarini RJ: Changes in prevalence, severity and recovery in tardive dyskinesia with age. Archives of General Psychiatry 37:1368–1373, 1980

24. Campbell A, Baldessarini RJ: Effects of maturation and aging on behavioral responses to haloperidol in the rat. Psychopharmacology 73:219–222, 1981

25. Laska E, Varga E, Wanderling J, et al: Patterns of psychotropic drug use for schizophrenia. Diseases of the Nervous System 34:294–305, 1973

26. Chouinard G, Jones B, Annable L, et al: Sex differences and tardive dyskinesia (ltr). American Journal of Psychiatry 137:507, 1980

27. Gordon J, Borison R, Diamond B: Modulation of dopamine receptor sensitivity by estrogen. Biological Psychiatry 15:389–396, 1980

28. Simpson GM, Varga E, Lee JH, et al: Tardive dyskinesia and psychotropic drug history. Psychopharmacology 58:117–124, 1978

29. Smith HM, Oswald WT, Kucharski T, et al: Tardive dyskinesia: age and sex differences in hospitalized schizophrenics. Psychopharmacology 58:207–211, 1978

30. Yassa R, Nair V: Incidence of tardive dyskinesia in an outpatient population. Psychosomatics 25:479–481, 1984

31. Baldessarini RJ: Clinical and epidemiologic aspects of tardive dyskinesia. Journal of Clinical Psychiatry 46:8–13, 1985

32. Gualtieri CT, Quade D, Hicks RE, et al: Tardive dyskinesia and other clinical consequences of neuroleptic treatment in children and adolescents. American Journal of Psychiatry 141:20–23, 1984

33. Pryce IG, Edward H: Persistent oral dyskinesia in female mental hospital patients. British Journal of Psychiatry 112:983–987, 1966

34. Crane GE: High dose of trifluoperazine and tardive dyskinesia. Archives of Neurology 22:176–180, 1970

35. Crane GE, Sneets RA: Tardive dyskinesia and drug therapy in geriatric patients. British Journal of Psychiatry 30:341–343, 1976

36. Ogita K, Yogi G, Itoh H: Comparative analysis of persistent dyskinesia of long-term usage with neuroleptics in France and in Japan. Folia Psychiatrica et Neurologica 29:315–320, 1975

37. Kane JM, Rifkin A, Woerner M, et al: Low-dose neuroleptic treatment of outpatient schizophrenics. Archives of General Psychiatry 40:893–896, 1983

38. Kane JM, Smith JM: Tardive dyskinesia: prevalence and risk factors, 1959 to 1979. Archives of General Psychiatry 39:473–481, 1982

39. Jeste D: Prevention, management and treatment of tardive dyskinesia. Journal of Clinical Psychiatry 46:14–18, 1985

40. Mukherjee S, Rosen AM, Cardenas C, et al: Tardive dyskinesia in psychiatric outpatients: a study of prevalence and association with demographic, clinical, and drug history variables. Archives of General Psychiatry 39:466–469, 1982

41. Simpson GM, Pi EH, Sramek JJ: Current status of tardive dyskinesia. Journal of Psychiatric Treatment and Evaluation 5:127–133, 1983

42. Gee S, Mesard L: Psychiatric Drug Study, Part I: Psychiatric Ward Unit Study. Office of the Controllers Monograph No 9. Washington, DC, US Veterans Administration, 1979

43. Csernansky JG, Grabowski K, Cervantes J, et al: Fluphenazine decanoate and tardive dyskinesia: a possible association. American Journal of Psychiatry 138:1362–1365, 1981

44. Goldberg SC, Shenoy RS, Julius D, et al: Does long-acting injectable neuroleptic protect against tardive dyskinesia? Psychopharmacology Bulletin 18:177–179, 1982

45. Perris C, Dimitrijevic P, Jacobsson L, et al: Tardive dyskinesia in psychiatric patients treated with neuroleptics. British Journal of Psychiatry 135:509–514, 1979

46. Jeste DV, Linnoila M, Wagner RL, et al: Serum neuroleptic concentrations and tardive dyskinesia. Psychopharmacology 75:377–380, 1982

47. Csernansky JG, Kaplan J, Holman CA, et al: Serum neuroleptic activity, protection, and tardive dyskinesia in schizophrenic outpatients. Psychopharmacology 81:115–118, 1983

48. Crane GE: Pseudoparkinsonism and tardive dyskinesia. Archives of Neurology 27:426–430, 1972

49. Gerlach J: The relationship between parkinsonism and tardive dyskinesia. American Journal of Psychiatry 134:781–784, 1977

50. Fann WE, Lake CR: On the coexistence of parkinsonism and tardive dyskinesia. Diseases of the Nervous System 35:325–326, 1974

51. Defraites EG Jr, Davis KL, Berger PA: Coexisting tardive dyskinesia and parkinsonism: a case report. Biological Psychiatry 12:147–152, 1977

52. Chouinard G, Annable L, Ross-Chouinard A, et al: Ethopropazine and benztropine in neuroleptic-induced parkinsonism. Journal of Clinical Psychiatry 41:147–152, 1959

53. Turek I, Kurland AA, Hanlon TE, et

al: Tardive dyskinesia: its relationship to neuroleptic and antiparkinson drugs. British Journal of Psychiatry 121:605–612, 1972

54. Kiloh LG, Smith SJ, Williams SE: Antiparkinson drugs as causal agents in tardive dyskinesia. Medical Journal of Australia 2:591–593, 1973

55. Chouinard G, De Montigny C, Annable L: Tardive dyskinesia and antiparkinsonian medication. American Journal of Psychiatry 136:228–229, 1979

56. Gardos G, Cole JO: Tardive dyskinesia and anticholinergic drugs. American Journal of Psychiatry 140:200–202, 1983

57. Cunningham Owens DG, Johnston EC, Frith CD: Spontaneous involuntary disorders of movement: their prevalence, severity, and distribution in chronic schizophrenics with and without treatment with neuroleptics. Archives of General Psychiatry 39:452–461, 1982

58. Tardive dyskinesia. Report of the American Psychiatric Association Task Force on Later Neurological Effects of Antipsychotic Drugs. Washington, DC, American Psychiatric Association, 1979

59. Klawans HL: The pharmacology of tardive dyskinesia. American Journal of Psychiatry 130:82–86, 1973

60. Kazamatsuri H, Chien C-P, Cole J: Long-term treatment of tardive dyskinesia with haloperidol and tetrabenazine. American Journal of Psychiatry 130:479–483, 1973

61. Claveria L, Teychenne P, Calne D, et al: Tardive dyskinesia treated with pimozide. Journal of the Neurological Sciences 24:393–401, 1975

62. Kebabia J, Calne D: Multiple receptors for dopamine. Nature 277:93–96, 1978

63. Casey D, Gerlach J, Simmelsgaard H: Sulpiride in tardive dyskinesia. Psychopharmacology 66:73–77, 1979

64. Casey D, Gerlach J: Oxiperomide in tardive dyskinesia. Journal of Neurology, Neurosurgery, and Psychiatry 43:264–267, 1980

65. White FJ, Wang RY: Differential effects of classical and atypical antipsychotic drugs on A9 and A10 dopamine neurons. Science 221:1054–1056, 1983

66. Meltzer HY, Luchins DJ: Effect of clozapine in severe tardive dyskinesia: a case report. Journal of Clinical Psychopharmacology 4:286–287, 1984

67. Sternberg DE: Lithium prevents adaptation of brain dopamine systems to haloperidol in schizophrenic patients. Psychiatry Research 10:79, 1983

68. Simpson GM, Branchey MH, Lee JM, et al: Lithium in tardive dyskinesia. Pharmakopsychiatria 9:76–80, 1976

69. Yassa R, Archer J, Cordozo S: The long-term effect of lithium carbonate on tardive dyskinesia. Canadian Journal of Psychiatry 29:36–37, 1984

70. Godwin-Austin R, Clark T: Persistent phenothiazine dyskinesia treated with tetrabenazine. British Medical Journal 4:25–26, 1971

71. Kazamatsuri H, Chien C-P, Cole J: Treatment of tardive dyskinesia. Archives of General Psychiatry 27:824–827, 1972

72. Baldessarini RJ, Tarsy D: Tardive dyskinesia, in Psychopharmacology: A Generation of Progress. Edited by Lipton M, DiMascio A, Killam KF. New York, Raven, 1978

73. Donatelli A, Geisen L, Feuer E: Case report of adverse effect of reserpine on tardive dyskinesia. American Journal of Psychiatry 140:239–240, 1983

74. Bjorndal N, Casey DE, Gerlach J, et al: The effect of levodopa in tardive dyskinesia, in Phenothiazines and Structurally Related Drugs: Basic and Clinical Studies. Edited by Usdin E, Eckert H, Forrest I. Amsterdam, Elsevier–North Holland, 1980

75. Jeste DV, DeLisi LE, Saleman S, et al: A biochemical study of tardive dyskinesia in young male patients. Psychiatric Research 4:327–331, 1981

76. Wagner RL, Jeste DL, Phelps BH, et al: Enzyme studies in tardive dyskinesia. Journal of Clinical Psychopharmacology 2:312–314, 1982

77. Davis KL, Berger P: Pharmacological investigations of the cholinergic imbalance hypothesis of movement disorders and psychosis. Biological Psychiatry 13:23–49, 1978

78. Ingram NA, Newgreen DB: The use of tacrine for tardive dyskinesia. American Journal of Psychiatry 140:1629–1631, 1983

79. Nasrallah HA, Dunner FJ, Smith RE, et al: Variable clinical response to choline in tardive dyskinesia. Psychological Medicine 14:697–700, 1984

80. Jackson IV, Nuttall EA, Ibe IO, et al: Treatment of tardive dyskinesia with lecithin. American Journal of Psychiatry 136:1458–1460, 1979

81. Perez-Cruet J, Menendez I, Alvarez-Ghersi J, et al: Double-blind study of lecithin in the treatment of persistent tardive dyskinesia. Boletin Asociacion Medica de Puerto Rico 73:531–537, 1981

82. Growdon J: Lecithin can suppress tardive dyskinesia. New England Journal of Medicine 298:1029, 1978

83. Growdon J: Choline and lecithin administration to patients with tardive dyskinesia. Canadian Journal of Neurological Sciences 6:89, 1979

84. Gardos G, Cole JO, Rapkin RM, et al: Anticholinergic challenge and neuroleptic withdrawal: changes in dyskinesia and symptom measures. Archives of General Psychiatry 41:1030–1035, 1984

85. Singh MM, Becker RE, Pitman RK, et al: Sustained improvement in tardive dyskinesia with diazepam: indirect evidence for corticolimbic involvement.

Brain Research Bulletin 11:179–185, 1983

86. Weber SS, Dufresne RL, Becker RE, et al: Diazepam in tardive dyskinesia. Drug Intelligence and Clinical Pharmacy 17:523–527, 1983

87. Wolf ME, Keener S, Mathis P, et al: Phenylethylamine-like properties of baclofen. Neuropsychobiology 9:219–222, 1983

88. Casey DE, Hammerstad JP: Sodium valproate in tardive dyskinesia. Journal of Clinical Psychiatry 40:483–485, 1979

89. Tamminga CA, Crayton JW, Chase TN: Improvement in tardive dyskinesia after muscimol therapy. Archives of General Psychiatry 36:595–598, 1979

90. Korsgaard S, Casey DE, Gerlach L: Effect of gamma-vinyl GABA in tardive dyskinesia. Psychiatry Research 8:261–269, 1983

91. Nishikawa T, Tanaka M, Koga I, et al: Combined treatment of tardive dyskinesia with clonidine and neuroleptics: a follow-up study of three cases for three years. Psychopharmacology 80:374–375, 1983

92. Nishikawa T, Tanaka M, Tsuda A, et al: Clonidine therapy for tardive dyskinesia and related syndromes. Clinical Neuropharmacology 7:239–245, 1984

93. Jeste DV, Potkin SG, Sinha S, et al: Tardive dyskinesia: reversible and persistent. Archives of General Psychiatry 36:585–590, 1979

94. Branchey M, Branchey L: Patterns of psychotropic drug use and tardive dyskinesia. Journal of Clinical Psychopharmacology 4:41–45, 1984

95. Glazer WM, Moore DC, Schooler NR, et al: Tardive dyskinesia: a discontinuation study. Archives of General Psychiatry 41:623–627, 1984

96. McInnis M, Petursson H: Withdrawal of trihexyphenidyl. Acta Psychiatrica Scandinavica 71:297–303, 1985

97. Chouinard G, Bradwejn J, Annable L, et al: Withdrawal symptoms after long-term treatment with low-potency neuroleptics. Journal of Clinical Psychiatry 45:500–502, 1984

Intermittent Neuroleptic Therapy and Tardive Dyskinesia: A Literature Review

Morris B. Goldman, M.D.
Daniel J. Luchins, M.D.

Many authorities advocate neuroleptic-free periods for patients on chronic neuroleptics as a means of reducing the incidence or severity of tardive dyskinesia. This practice continues, despite the absence of any controlled clinical studies showing that intermittent therapy reduces the incidence or progression of tardive dyskinesia. After reviewing the pertinent clinical and animal literature, the authors conclude that there are few data to support the use of intermittent therapy as a means of reducing tardive dyskinesia and, in fact, evidence suggests it may increase the risk of persistent tardive dyskinesia.

The brief interruption of chronic neuroleptic therapy (drug holidays) was first vigorously advocated by Ayd in 1965 (1). After reviewing evidence that most patients do not relapse immediately after discontinuation of neuroleptic therapy, he described his expe-

Dr. Goldman is a resident in the department of psychiatry and Dr. Luchins is associate professor in the department of psychiatry at the University of Chicago Pritzker School of Medicine. Address correspondence to Dr. Goldman, Department of Psychiatry, University of Chicago, Box 411, 5841 South Maryland Avenue, Chicago, Illinois 60637. The authors thank Daniel X. Freedman, M.D., Herbert Y. Meltzer, M.D., and Runae Hartfield for assistance with this manuscript.

rience with two types of drug holidays. In one group of patients a "never-on-Sunday" policy of maintenance neuroleptic therapy was initiated, which in some cases was extended to a two- or three-day drug holiday. Another group was maintained on a program of three weeks on medication and one week off, with a few patients having the drug-free period extended to two, three, or four weeks.

Ayd noted that although some patients had to be returned to medication before the end of the holiday, none of the patients had a serious relapse. He suggested that such intermittent therapy might reduce the "possible risk of toxic effects from continuous chemical assault on the body," including the risk of tardive dyskinesia (2).

During the intervening years no definitive means of treating or preventing tardive dyskinesia has been described; thus many authorities (3–6) continue to advocate intermittent therapy for inpatient and selected outpatient populations. For instance, the 1980 American Psychiatric Association task force on tardive dyskinesia recommended that neuroleptics be discontinued slowly (a 10-percent decrease every three days), followed by a drug-free period lasting a minimum of two weeks (6). The task force advised that this procedure be carried out at least once, and preferably twice, each year.

Since there are no prospective studies comparing the incidence or severity of tardive dyskinesia among patients maintained on intermittent therapy versus those on continuous therapy, advocates of intermittent therapy have based their support on the following logi-

cal grounds. First, intermittent therapy reduces cumulative neuroleptic dosage, thereby at least retarding the development of tardive dyskinesia (1,7,8). Second, it facilitates the early detection of tardive dyskinesia that might be reversible and thus helps to prevent persistent tardive dyskinesia (3,6). Third, it allows dopaminergic neurons to "down regulate," thus reducing the development of supersensitive dopamine receptors (5,6). Fourth, it enables the clinician to evaluate the need for antipsychotic medication and will at least help him effectively establish a minimum dosage (6,9).

Whereas Ayd emphasized the first rationale for instituting frequent drug holidays, recently authorities have tended to emphasize the latter three rationales and have recommended less frequent, but still regular, neuroleptic-free intervals. We will review the evidence that intermittent therapy reduces the risk of tardive dyskinesia and then examine the available literature for each of the four rationales. We will restrict our attention to clinical reports of drug-free periods of at least two weeks' duration since this is the minimum period currently recommended. The extensive literature on briefer drug holidays lasting two to four days has been reviewed elsewhere (10).

Clinical studies of intermittent therapy

We are aware of only one prospective study examining the effects of intermittent therapy on tardive dyskinesia. Gibson (11) discontinued neuroleptic therapy among 15 patients with tardive dyskinesia and observed them until the tardive dyskinesia remitted. During this period of unknown length, six patients had a psychotic relapse while still exhibiting tardive dyskinesia.

Among the remaining nine patients, however, the tardive dyskinesia remitted. These nine patients were then treated with depot neuroleptics, with one- to two-month drug-free intervals every three or four months. Over the 30 months of the study, only one patient had a recurrence of tardive dyskinesia. Since the author had noted a much higher recurrence rate of tardive dyskinesia in other patients treated continuously with neuroleptics, including 4 mg of pimozide daily or a halving of the previous depot-neuroleptic dosage, he suggested that intermittent therapy might have a prophylactic effect.

However, the study has numerous shortcomings, including the absence of a control group on continuous neuroleptic therapy, no rating scales for tardive dyskinesia, and no mention of dosage before or during intermittent therapy. Moreover, it is unclear whether the patients actually were drug-free since depot neuroleptics can be detected in the serum up to 12 weeks after an injection (12); in this study the longest period between injections was eight weeks.

In a retrospective study Jeste and associates (13) attempted to determine which variables distinguished patients with persistent tardive dyskinesia from those with reversible tardive dyskinesia. They studied 21 patients with tardive dyskinesia who were maintained without neuroleptics for four to 13 months. The nine whose tardive dyskinesia remained unabated were said to have persistent tardive dyskinesia, while those whose tardive dyskinesia remitted were said to have reversible tardive dyskinesia. Jeste and associates found that the patients with persistent tardive dyskinesia had undergone more neuroleptic-free periods of two months or longer than had either those with reversible tardive dyskinesia or control subjects who did not have tardive dyskinesia.

Because the patients with persistent tardive dyskinesia also had a significantly longer exposure to neuroleptics, had been neuroleptic-free a longer period of time, had been ill longer, and had tardive dyskinesia longer, the authors carried out a stepwise discriminant function analysis to identify the most important explanatory variable.

Cumulative dosage may not be an important factor in the development of tardive dyskinesia in chronic patients, the very population for which intermittent therapy is proposed.

---

able. The results showed that the number of drug-free periods was the variable that best differentiated persistent from reversible tardive dyskinesia, correctly classifying 76 percent of the patients.

One of the shortcomings of the study is its retrospective nature. Because the patients were not randomly assigned to receive intermittent or continuous treatment, it is unclear if the two groups are otherwise identical. For instance, it has been reported that patients with affective illness, who are more likely to receive medication intermittently, may also be predisposed to develop tardive dyskinesia (14).

Although Jeste and associates report a similar distribution of diagnoses in both groups, it is widely recognized that diagnostic categories may group together heterogeneous populations and these might not be equally distributed. Furthermore, in light of recent evidence that tardive dyskinesia may remit after two to five years (15), Jeste and associates' follow-up period was inadequate to assess reversibility. And, finally, a discriminant function analysis might not be appropriate for this small sample size (16).

The finding of Jeste and associates is supported by Degkwitz (17), who reported that drug interruptions (length unspecified) were twice as common in patients who developed tardive dyskinesia than in patients without tardive dyskinesia. Details of this finding have not been published, however. There is also another study that might contradict the findings of Jeste and associates. Crane (18) found no relationship between the percentage of time patients were neuroleptic-free and the prevalence of tardive dyskinesia in a sample of 669 inpatients.

All of these clinical studies address somewhat different issues. Gibson (11) instituted intermittent therapy to assess whether it lowered the recurrence rate of reversible tardive dyskinesia, and Jeste and associates (13) identified the variables that differed in patients with reversible or persistent tardive dyskinesia. In contrast, Degkwitz (17) and Crane (18) examined the effect of drug interruptions and percent of time drug-free on the incidence of tardive dyskinesia, but did not examine reversibility. Comparisons between these studies are difficult to make; clearly, controlled prospective studies are needed.

Cumulative dosage and intermittent therapy

As mentioned earlier, one of the rationales for intermittent neuroleptic therapy is that it might decrease the risk of tardive dyskinesia by reducing the cumulative neuroleptic dosage. However, the relationship of cumulative dosage to tardive dyskinesia is far from clear. This question has been thoroughly reviewed by Kane and Smith (16), who note that only four of the 18 controlled studies show a significant positive relationship between cumulative dosage and tardive dyskinesia.

Furthermore, positive studies involve samples with relatively low cumulative drug exposure. The authors go on to suggest, as have others (19), that cumulative dosage is probably important only in the first few years of neuroleptic therapy. Thus cumulative dosage may not be an important factor in the development of tardive dyskinesia in chronic patients, the very population for which intermittent therapy is proposed.

Notwithstanding the unresolved question of whether cumulative dosage is related to the development of tardive dyskinesia, several authors have attempted to demonstrate that intermittent therapy is an effective way of reducing cumulative exposure. Pyke and Seeman (20) instituted a program of six-week drug-free periods every six months for 14 chronic schizophrenic patients. There were a total of 24 drug-free periods over the one to two and a half years patients participated in the study.

Of the 14 patients, ten achieved a reduced neuroleptic maintenance dose; of these ten, four became drug-free. However, three of the patients ended up taking higher doses than originally prescribed. Moreover, eight experienced a recurrence of schizophrenic symptoms at some time during the study, and four required rehospitalization. Without a control group, it is impossible to determine whether a comparable reduction in dosage could have been achieved with less morbidity using continuous therapy.

There is also evidence that extended drug-free periods may not necessarily lead to reduced neuroleptic dosages. Branchey and associates (9) carried out a double-blind controlled study of 21 patients who were gradually withdrawn from neuroleptics over 18 weeks. At six-month follow-up, they were compared with 11 patients who had been continuously maintained on neuroleptics. When patients withdrawn from neuroleptics showed signs of relapse, their medication was restarted and gradually increased as needed.

During the 42 weeks of the study, two of the 11 (18 percent) continuous-therapy patients showed signs of deterioration compared with 16 of the 21 (76 percent) intermittent-therapy patients. Thirteen of the 16 patients showed symptoms after drugs were completely withdrawn. When returned to drug therapy, eight of these 13 required an equal or greater neuroleptic dosage than they had received before entering the study. On the other hand, five of the 21 (24 percent) intermittent-therapy patients managed to remain drug-free. These five patients were all over 50 years old and had been on low doses of neuroleptics.

Thus, although routine drug withdrawal or holidays might reduce cumulative dosage and identify patients who do not require medication, these procedures do not guarantee such an outcome. A significant proportion of patients end up requiring similar or greater dosages. Moreover, the rate of relapse may be high. Studies (21,22) showing that stable patients can be maintained on very low doses of neuroleptics (75 to 150 mg of chlorpromazine or 1.25 to 5 mg of fluphenazine decanoate) suggest that safer alternatives may exist.

Intermittent therapy and early detection

Another rationale for intermittent therapy is that it will allow for early detection of tardive dyskinesia (6,23), since even low dosages of neuroleptics can suppress tardive dyskinesia symptoms (19,22). It is assumed that after early detection neuroleptics can be reduced or stopped, which in turn might reduce the severity of tardive dyskinesia.

We are aware of only one study that has specifically examined patients whose tardive dyskinesia could be identified only after drug withdrawal. Carpenter and associates (24) withdrew 52 ambulatory schizophrenic patients from medication for four weeks; none of the patients showed signs of tardive dyskinesia before drug withdrawal. During this drug-free period 14 patients (27 percent) manifested tardive dyskinesia. The authors tried to maintain the patients drug-free to allow their tardive dyskinesia to remit, but all of the patients needed to be restarted on medication. The most disturbing finding was that, even after the patients were returned to neuroleptics, all but one continued to exhibit tardive dyskinesia. Thus, for this group of patients, drug withdrawal was not a good means of preventing tardive dyskinesia.

Dopamine-receptor sensitivity

In order to assess the contention that drug holidays allow dopamine receptors to "down regulate," thereby retarding supersensitivity, one must examine animal models of tardive dyskinesia. The relevance of animal models of tardive dyskinesia to the human patient has been questioned because the behavioral appearance, time course, persistence, and temporal relation to neuroleptic treatment of dyskinetic movements often differs in experimental animals and chronically psychotic patients (19).

Furthermore, several of the animal models are based on the unproven hypothesis that dopamine supersensitivity in the striatum causes tardive dyskinesia. While it is widely accepted that this hypersensitivity occurs with chronic neuroleptic treatment, its relation to tardive dyskinesia is unknown (19).

The animal model with the greatest similarity to tardive dyskinesia in man was developed by Kovacic and Domino (25). A syndrome resembling tardive dyskinesia was noted in three cebus apella monkeys following drug discontinuation after one year of fluphenazine enanthate injections (up to 3.2 mg/kg biweekly). One monkey was given three additional biweekly injections of 3.2 mg/kg of fluphenazine enanthate during the first two months after drugs were initially stopped and then again three and a half months later.

After each additional treatment course, the tardive dyskinesia became more severe and took longer to reverse. The authors concluded that intermittent therapy might change reversible tardive dyskinesia into a persistent form. However, since only one monkey was studied, no continuous-treatment control was available, and persistent tardive dyskinesia was never noted, these conclusions are speculative. Nevertheless, the findings raise the possibility that intermittent therapy might aggravate tardive dyskinesia.

Jeste and associates (26) treated rats with 1.25 mg/kg of haloperidol daily for 44 days or 1.5 mg/kg for three 12-day periods interrupted by four-day drug-free periods. The response of these animals to 2 mg/kg of amphetamine was assessed before treatment and again six and ten days after treatment. Both groups of animals showed an equal increase in amphetamine-induced locomotor activity and stereotypy relative to pretreatment levels. A possible flaw in this design is that drug-free periods lasting four days may not have been sufficient to produce a drug-free state in the animals, considering the 12- to 22-hour half-life of haloperidol (27).

Studying monkeys, Weiss and Santelli (28) reported that episodes of abnormal movements, developing one to eight hours after drug consumption, occurred more rapidly and reliably when the animals received an equivalent cumulative dosage of haloperidol weekly as opposed to daily. Although the authors theorized that these abnormal movements might provide a model of tardive dyskinesia, the movements' rapid onset after drug administration and subsequent disappearance suggest that this is not the case. The described pattern more closely resembles that of the acute dyskinesia.

A different approach to this question has been taken by Bannet and associates (29), who compared changes in dopamine receptor binding in mice caudate after continuous and intermittent haloperidol therapy. They found no difference between the groups. To the extent that a short-term increase in dopamine binding might be a relevant model of the pathophysiology of tardive dyskinesia, the study does not support intermittent therapy.

Feasibility and risks

The potential benefits of intermittent therapy need to be balanced against its associated morbidity. As portrayed by Shenoy and associates (30), intermittent therapy is quite benign. They examined relapse rate and abnormal movements in 31 chronic schizophrenic patients who had been receiving fluphenazine decanoate for at least two years. Seventeen patients underwent two six-week drug holidays, while 14 patients continued on medication.

Both experimental and control-group patients remained in remission, and there was no overall increase in abnormal movements in either group. However, although the group of 17 underwent a drug holiday, there is reason to believe they were not drug-free. As mentioned previously, fluphenazine decanoate can be detected in serum up to three months after the last injection (11).

Olson and Peterson (31) noted a less favorable outcome with intermittent therapy in a chronically hospitalized population. Patients were randomly assigned to one of two treatment regimens: drug therapy alternating monthly with placebo and drug therapy alternating monthly with no therapy.

Olson and Peterson noted a relapse rate of 29 percent in the placebo group and 85 percent in the no-therapy group over the six months of the study. Because of the profound effect of placebo, the authors subsequently crossed-over the two intermittent-therapy groups for a one-month period of either placebo or no therapy. They then noted a relapse rate of 14 percent in the placebo group and 43 percent in the group that received no therapy.

This finding, highlighting the importance of expectations and intolerance to change, is supported by the results of Lesser and Friedman's study (32). Forty percent of the 52 chronic schizophrenic patients these authors surveyed felt that they could not, or would not, tolerate even a one-week drug holiday. Many clinicians also report that chronic schizophrenic patients and their families deal poorly with abrupt changes in treatment and vastly prefer unchanging regimens.

Herz and associates (33) report probably the most compelling evidence that drug discontinuation may be feasible. However, their program is not really one of intermittent therapy with fixed periods of drug treatment and drug withdrawal, but rather one of targeted drug treatment aimed at early detection of prodromal signs of psychosis. They attempted to discontinue the medication of 19 stable schizophrenic outpatients over a period of eight weeks. This study was conducted in the context of an active outpatient program that provided weekly group sessions, counseling about the prodromal signs of relapse, and treating psychiatrists who could be reached by telephone on a 24-hour basis.

Five patients experienced prodromal signs during the initial drug withdrawal and were dropped from the study. Of the remaining 14 patients, five remained drug-free throughout the approximately eight months of the study. Five others who had prodromal symptoms were briefly returned to medication and then were again successfully withdrawn. Four others either dropped out or their conditions deteriorated so that medication could not be stopped again. Thus the program was at least partially successful for ten of the original 19 patients.

This study demonstrated that with an active outpatient support program some chronic schizophrenic patients can be maintained drug-free for certain lengths of time. The cost of this outcome in possibly increased morbidity cannot be estimated without a similarly treated group of patients who received continuous medication. Furthermore, the relevance of this approach to intermittent drug therapy remains unclear.

Conclusion

After reviewing the evidence, we found little support for the view that intermittent neuroleptic therapy might reduce the incidence or severity of tardive dyskinesia. In fact, evidence exists that intermittent therapy might be associated with an increased risk of persistent tardive dyskinesia (13), conversion of latent tardive dyskinesia into a persistent form (24), and increased dopaminergic sensitivity (25). Furthermore, intermittent therapy can lead to increased, not decreased, maintenance dosage (9) and may be associated with a relatively high rate of relapse (20,31).

Clearly, controlled studies are needed to establish the benefits of intermittent therapy. Until that time, however, intermittent neuroleptic therapy cannot be advocated as a means of retarding the development or progression of tardive dyskinesia.

References

1. Ayd FJ: Drug holidays: intermittent pharmacotherapy for psychiatric patients. International Drug Therapy Newsletter 8:1–3, 1966
2. Ayd FJ: Drug holidays: intermittent pharmacotherapy for psychiatric patients. Medical Science, 1967, pp 59–62
3. Crane GE: Prevention and management of tardive dyskinesia. American Journal of Psychiatry 129:466–467, 1972
4. Tardive dyskinesia (edtl). Lancet 2:447–449, 1979
5. Klawans HL, Goetz CG, Perlik S: Tardive dyskinesia: review and update. American Journal of Psychiatry 137:900–907, 1980
6. Tardive dyskinesia: summary of a task force report of the APA. American Journal of Psychiatry 137:1163–1172, 1980
7. Marder SR, van Kammen DP, Docherty JP, et al: Predicting drug-free improvement in schizophrenic psychosis. Archives of General Psychiatry 36:1080–1085, 1979
8. Lehmann HE: Psychopharmacological treatment of schizophrenia. Schizophrenia Bulletin 13:27–45, 1975
9. Branchey MH, Branchey LB, Richardson MA: Effects of gradual decrease and discontinuation of neuroleptics on clinical condition and tardive dyskinesia. Psychopharmacology Bulletin 1:118–120, 1981
10. Davis JM, Erickson SE, Tsai CC: Antipsychotic drugs: some current concepts. Illinois Department of Mental Health Journal of Research 2:24–30, 1974
11. Gibson AL: Effect of drug holidays on tardive dyskinesia, in Phenothiazines and Structurally Related Drugs: Basic and Clinical Studies. Edited by Usdin E, Forrest IS. New York, Elsevier-North Holland, 1980

12. McCreadie RG, Dingwall JM, Wiles DH, et al: Intermittent pimozide versus fluphenazine decanoate as maintenance therapy in chronic schizophrenia. British Journal of Psychiatry 137:510–517, 1980
13. Jeste DV, Potkin DG, Sinha S, et al: Tardive dyskinesia: reversible and persistent. Archives of General Psychiatry 36:585–590, 1979
14. Rosenbaum KM, Niven RG, Hanson MP, et al: Tardive dyskinesia: relationship with affective disorder. Diseases of the Nervous System 38:423–427, 1977
15. Casey DE, Toenniessen L: Tardive dyskinesia: what is the natural history? International Drug Therapy Newsletter 18:13–16, 1983
16. Kane JM, Smith JM: Tardive dyskinesia: prevalence and risk factors, 1959 to 1979. Archives of General Psychiatry 39:473–481, 1982
17. Degkwitz R: Extrapyramidal motor disorders following long-term treatment with neuroleptic drugs, in Psychotropic Drugs and Dysfunction of the Basal Ganglia. Edited by Crane GE, Gardner R. Public Health Service Publication 1938. Rockville, Md, National Institute of Mental Health, 1969
18. Crane GE: Factors predisposing to drug-induced neurologic effects, in The Phenothiazines and Structurally Related Drugs. Edited by Forrest IS, Carr CV, Usdin E. New York, Raven Press, 1974
19. Jeste DV, Wyatt RJ: Understanding and Treating Tardive Dyskinesia. New York, Guilford, 1982
20. Pyke J, Seeman MN: Neuroleptic-free intervals in the treatment of schizophrenia. American Journal of Psychiatry 138:1620–1621, 1981
21. Kane JM, Rifkin A, Quitkin F, et al: Low-dose fluphenazine decanoate in maintenance therapy of schizophrenia. Psychiatry Research 1:341–348, 1979
22. Lonowski DJ: Gradual reduction of neuroleptic medication among chronic schizophrenics. Acta Psychiatrica Scandinavica 57:97–102, 1972
23. Jeste DV, Wyatt RJ: Therapeutic strategies against tardive dyskinesia. Archives of General Psychiatry 39:803–816, 1982
24. Carpenter WT, Rey AC, Stephens JH: Covert dyskinesia in ambulatory schizophrenics. Lancet 2:212–213, 1980
25. Kovacic B, Domino E: A monkey model of tardive dyskinesia: evidence that tardive dyskinesia may turn into irreversible tardive dyskinesia. Journal of Clinical Psychopharmacology 2:305–307, 1982
26. Jeste DV, Stoff DS, Potkin SG, et al: Amphetamine sensitivity and tardive dyskinesia: an animal model. Indian Journal of Psychiatry 21:362–369, 1979
27. Frosman A, Ohman R: On the pharmacokinetics of haloperidol. Nordisk-Psykiatrisk Tidsokrift 28:441–448, 1974

28. Weiss B, Santelli S: Dyskinesia evoked in monkeys by weekly administration of haloperidol. Science 200:799–801, 1978
29. Bannet J, Belmaker RH, Ebstein RP: The effect of drug holidays in an animal model of tardive dyskinesia. Psychopharmacology 69:223–224, 1980
30. Shenoy RS, Sadler AG, Goldberg SC, et al: Effects of a six-week drug holiday on symptom status, relapse, and tardive dyskinesia in chronic schizophrenics. Journal of Clinical Psychopharmacology 1:141–145, 1981
31. Olson GW, Peterson DB: Intermittent chemotherapy for chronic psychiatric inpatients. Journal of Nervous and Mental Disorders 134:145–149, 1962
32. Lesser IM, Friedman CTH: Attitudes toward medication change among chronically impaired psychiatric patients. American Journal of Psychiatry 138:801–803, 1981
33. Herz MI, Syzmanski HV, Simon JC: Intermittent medication for stable schizophrenic outpatients. American Journal of Psychiatry 139:918–919, 1982

Movement Disorders in the Psychiatric Patient

Daniel A. Moros, M.D.
Melvin D. Yahr, M.D.

Abnormal movements or postures often present a diagnostic and therapeutic challenge to the psychiatrist or neurologist. The authors review pertinent anatomy and physiology of disorders of the extrapyramidal system, suggest aspects of the clinical history and examination particularly important for diagnosis, and describe a range of abnormal movements. They review several syndromes in which abnormalities of behavior and movement may occur together, including Huntington's chorea, Wilson's disease, Parkinson's disease, and tardive dyskinesia.

The link between motor behavior and psychological state is an intimate one. Our faces often automatically express sadness, concern, and joy even when we successfully restrain our speech or action. Anxiety is often accompanied by motor restlessness. Tension and the performance of relatively simple intellectual tasks tend to exacerbate preexisting abnormalities of motor activity such as tremor and dyskinesia. It is not surprising that there exist a variety of neurologic syndromes manifesting abnormalities of movement and behavior, or that we find an overlap between the pharmacologic agents used to con-

Dr. Moros is assistant professor of clinical neurology and Dr. Yahr is chairman of the department of neurology at Mount Sinai School of Medicine, 1 Gustave Levy Place, New York, New York 10029.

trol mood and behavior and those that either exacerbate or relieve movement disorders.

The patient with abnormal movements or postures often presents a diagnostic and therapeutic challenge for the psychiatrist and neurologist. Patients with disorders such as tics or focal dystonias may be referred to the psychiatrist because the abnormal motor behavior is presumed to be of psychological origin. Patients with progressive neurologic syndromes such as Huntington's chorea or Wilson's disease may present with prominent behavioral abnormalities and relatively inconspicuous abnormal movements. And in the patient treated with neuroleptics for psychotic, impulsive, or agitated behavior, the appearance of abnormal involuntary movements may raise the question of drug effect versus an evolving neurologic syndrome whose first manifestations are behavioral abnormalities.

The psychiatrist encountering a patient with abnormal involuntary movements will want to be confident that this symptom has been properly evaluated. We will review some of the anatomy and physiology most useful for understanding the movement disorders; aspects of the clinical history and examination most immediately relevant to the characterization of abnormal involuntary movements; types of abnormal movements; and several syndromes that often present complex and variable patterns of abnormal movements and behavior.

Anatomy and physiology

Disordered motor performance is a common characteristic of central nervous system (CNS) dysfunc-

tion. Lesions involving the corticospinal tracts are classically characterized by loss of power, spasticity, increased tendon reflexes, and a Babinski's sign, but may at times be manifested only by clumsiness of a limb and an otherwise normal examination. Lesions involving sensory pathways may also produce clumsy, uncoordinated movements. When proprioception is severely affected, an involved limb may fail to maintain a fixed posture, and "pseudo-athetoid" movements may result. Traditionally neurologists distinguish between lesions of the pyramidal system, the sensory systems, and the extrapyramidal system. The distinction is useful but should not blind the examiner to the fact that normal movements represent an integrated output of much of the nervous system.

There are a number of syndromes classified under the rubric "movement disorders" that are predominantly a reflection of dysfunction of the extrapyramidal system. This system can be roughly defined as a group of deep cerebral, brainstem, and cerebellar nuclei and their connections, including the corpus striatum, several thalamic nuclei, and the substantia nigra. Extrapyramidal dysfunction may produce difficulty in initiating movement, abnormalities of posture and muscle tone, and hyperkinetic or dyskinetic movements of the limbs, mouth, face, and trunk. The dyskinetic or hyperkinetic movements, which will be described later, include tic, chorea, dystonia, athetosis, myoclonus, hemiballismus, and tremor.

The detailed physiology of the interconnected nuclear masses constituting the extrapyramidal system is not yet known, but the last two decades have seen a remarkable growth in our knowledge of the pharmacology and biochemical anatomy of these areas (1). Of particular import is the demonstration that disturbances in neurotransmitter relationships occur in this region of the brain and underlie the production of symptoms. Hence Parkinson's disease is characterized by reduced dopamine levels in the corpus striatum as a result of loss of dopaminergic cells originating in the substantia nigra. A parkinsonian syndrome may also be produced by neuroleptic agents that block the striatal dopamine receptors. It appears that a dopaminergic receptor within the corpus striatum modulates (through postsynaptic inhibition) a cholinergic pathway.

Thus parkinsonism can be thought of as a reflection of decreased dopaminergic activity or increased cholinergic activity, and indeed parkinsonism may be ameliorated by dopaminergic agonists, dopamine precursors (L-dopa), and anticholinergic agents. In addition, L-dopa may exacerbate preexisting chorea and athetosis and will produce these movements in the patients with Parkinson's disease. At least some of the hyperkinetic syndromes may reflect "increased dopaminergic tone." Dopamine receptor blockers will reduce the frequency of chorea and chronic motor tics.

Clinical history and examination

Age of onset of abnormal movements is particularly important. Have symptoms been present from birth or early childhood? If so, the movements may be the result of an intrauterine insult or trauma at birth (cerebral palsy). Such injuries may be associated with mental retardation or the later development of behavioral problems. Also, movement disorders secondary to such brain damage are not necessarily stable. They often are worse between ages two and four and may then improve. A

clear history of progression of symptoms is important in distinguishing the symptomatic expression of a stable lesion from an active disease process (2).

Were abnormal movements first noticed after head trauma or an infectious illness? Both have been implicated in causing damage to

---

The age of onset of abnormal movements is especially important. A complete family history should be obtained. At times it is desirable for a physician to examine family members.

---

basal ganglia nuclei.

Is there a family history of similar movements? The family history may be deceptive. Family members may be anxious to deny the presence of a genetic disease. Also, the age of onset and the symptoms themselves may vary within a given family. Thus some family members may be minimally affected, and their abnormal movements may either go unrecognized by relatives or be thought of as personal idiosyncrasies rather than "symptoms." Symptoms appearing in later years tend to be discounted as secondary to aging. At times it is desirable for a physician to examine family members.

Similarly, a complete family history, with age of siblings, parents, aunts, uncles, and cousins, should be obtained. A history of consanguinity is important, as diseases such as Wilson's disease and dystonia musculorum deformans are autosomal recessive disorders and are thus more likely to occur when parents are related. Huntington's chorea and a variety of cerebellar or multisystem degenerations with dementia have autosomal dominant patterns of inheritance. In Huntington's chorea the neurologic syndrome is ultimately fully manifested in all affected family

members. In the cerebellar syndromes there may be *forme fruste* and variable penetrance (3). In Huntington's and cerebellar degenerations personality change may be the earliest expression of an ultimately obvious neurologic disease.

The geographic origin of the parents also should be determined. Some diseases are seen with greater frequency among specific groups—for example, dystonia musculorum deformans usually occurs in Eastern European Jews.

Is there a history of hyperthyroidism or autoimmune disease? Behavior change and choreiform movements are seen in both these conditions.

What medications or illicit drugs has the patient been taking? Chorea has been reported in association with phenytoin, oral contraceptives, neuroleptic agents, isoniazide, lithium, and amphetamines.

What other illnesses does the patient have? Intermittent neurologic dysfunction may be seen with sickle cell anemia, polycythemia, valvular heart disease, and atrial myxoma, among other conditions.

During the examination abnormal movements and postures should be carefully observed and described. Abnormal movements may be more apparent during the performance of directed activities and during stress. The patient should be observed while walking and while performing a variety of intellectual tasks such as simple calculations and spelling backward. Tremor should be observed with the limbs at rest, with the limbs held in a variety of sustained postures, and during active movement.

Many abnormal movements reflecting basal ganglia dysfunction are associated with other signs of basal ganglia disease. The physician should observe the patient's facial expressiveness; volume and intonation of voice; muscle tone in the limbs, neck, and trunk; arm swing while walking; and balance. Skeletal abnormalities such as scoliosis or high arches suggest an underlying neurologic disease.

Similarly, abnormalities of the optic fundi or extraocular movements will further confirm primary neurologic disease. Some abnormalities will alert the physician to specific diagnoses; for example, cytoid bodies seen by funduscopic examination suggest systemic lupus erythematosus, and Kayser-Fleischer rings seen by routine or slit-lamp examination of the cornea suggest Wilson's disease.

Types of abnormal movements

Several kinds of involuntary movements that the consultant may see in movement disorders are described here.

Tic refers to a brief, stereotyped, purposeless movement. Tics are usually, but not necessarily, rapid. They occur at irregular intervals, and their frequency may vary considerably throughout the day or over longer periods of time. The patient can often voluntarily suppress the tic, although characteristically he finds that to do so requires a great effort that cannot be sustained. Tics may be accompanied by a "sense of compulsion," but it is not clear whether this internal experience represents an associated phenomenon or an actual "psychic cause."

Tics may be accompanied by grunts or simple verbalizations; when they occur, the disorder is called Gilles de la Tourette syndrome. It is not clear whether Tourette's represents a discrete entity or designates one part of a spectrum comprising single and multiple tics. Compared with the general population, family members of patients with Tourette's show a higher incidence of chronic single and multiple tics without verbalization. The illness does not appear to remit spontaneously. The simple, transient tic of childhood usually remits within one year and does not require treatment (4).

Chorea refers to abnormal involuntary movements that are rapid, purposeless, and not stereotyped. When it is mild, chorea may be mistaken for restlessness or nervousness. Similarly, when confined to a single limb or joint, it may first be mistaken for a tic. (Again, a tic is more stereotyped.) When chorea is more severe, there may be prominent facial grimacing, darting movements of the tongue, and twitching or turning movements of the head, neck, limbs, and trunk.

Choreatic movements involving the larger muscles may disrupt voluntary movements and produce an uncoordinated, jerky appearance. Patients may be able to suppress the abnormal movements for brief periods of time, but will be unable to maintain a posture of an involved limb. A classic sign of chorea is the "milkmaid's grip." Here, when the patient is asked to maintain a firm grip on the examiner's hand, the patient's hand will alternately contract and relax.

Choreas can be subdivided into acute and chronic syndromes (5). Acute chorea may accompany almost any disease involving the CNS. It may be seen with vasculitis, arteriosclerotic disease, encephalitis, and hyperviscosity syndromes; during pregnancy (chorea gravidarum); and with the use of a variety of drugs including L-dopa, amphetamines, opiates, and phenytoin. Classic acute chorea of the Sydenham's variety is usually seen in children between ages five and 15 and is frequently associated with rheumatic fever. The condition is benign and usually subsides within six months. Chronic chorea may be seen with a variety of neurodegenerative diseases of which the most common is Huntington's chorea. This condition will be discussed in more detail below.

Dystonia refers to slow, sustained powerful turning or twisting movements of the limbs or trunk. When a contraction is maintained over long periods of time, abnormal or dystonic postures occur. Dystonias may be classified as focal, such as spasmodic torticollis, writer's cramp, or blepharospasm; segmental, with symptoms usually beginning in the neck or face and later involving one or both extremities; and generalized, such as dystonia musculorum deformans.

Dystonia may be secondary to a specific neurologic insult such as perinatal injury (cerebral palsy) or Wilson's disease. In such cases other neurologic findings are often evident. Dystonias may also appear sporadically or as an inherited disease, such as the autosomal recessive pattern of dystonia musculorum deformans seen in Ashkenazi Jews. Dystonia may be progressive or relatively stable and may vary over time, with periods of relatively greater or lesser symptomatic expression. The idiopathic focal dystonias tend to be nonprogressive and usually begin in adult life (6).

The generalized dystonias usually begin in childhood; often their earliest symptom is an inverted and extended posture of the ankle (7). Dystonia is often initially mistaken for a psychiatric symptom. The child with leg involvement may have difficulty walking or running and may vary his or her social behavior to mask an embarrassing disability.

The focal dystonias may seem quite peculiar. A good example is writer's cramp, which is a focal dystonia involving the dominant hand and wrist (8). It appears as an uncontrollably tense grip of a pen or pencil with flexion of the wrist and marked pressure of the point against the paper. There may be some jerking or choreatic movements superimposed on the dystonic posture. Other finely coordinated movements of the hand are usually normal.

Writer's cramp may vary with different postures of the trunk and shoulder girdle, and thus the affected individual may be able to write when standing at a blackboard but have great difficulty when sitting at a desk. This syndrome is usually nonprogressive, particularly when it first appears in adult life. On closer questioning the patient may reveal a history of always having gripped a pen or pencil tightly and always having found prolonged writing difficult.

A similar syndrome is sometimes found with musicians. We have seen violinists who have difficulty only in fingering the strings of their instrument. Such unique difficulties limited to a single activity without clear abnormalities of strength, sensation, or reflexes and without evidence of other abnormal movements often raise a suspicion of a conversion reaction. The pathological basis of such conditions is not known.

The treatment of focal dystonias is disappointing. Benzodiazepine compounds such as diazepam and clonazepam are often used. Carbamazepine has been reported to be useful in treating some children with idiopathic focal dystonia. More recently there have been reports of successful treatment with high doses of anticholinergic agents (9).

Athetosis refers to slow, writhing movements of the limbs. As in chorea, the movements are irregular, rather than patterned. If the movements are moderately fast, the term choreoathetosis is often used. Some writers refer to the slow movements of dystonic syndromes as athetosis and the abnormal postures as dystonia.

The physiologic distinction between chorea, athetosis, dystonic movements, and abnormal postures is not clear. All may be present in a single patient. There are, however, clear pharmacologic distinctions, as some drugs such as neuroleptics may reduce chorea but not significantly influence athetosis or dystonia. On the other hand, chronic treatment of Parkinson's disease with dopaminergic agents will produce all forms of abnormal movements and postures.

Myoclonus refers to rapid, sudden contraction of a muscle with movement of a joint. Myoclonus may be focal or generalized, may be rhythmic or arrhythmic, and may be stimulus-linked or occur spontaneously. Myoclonic jerks commonly occur in normal persons when they are falling asleep. They also occur in stage-two sleep and may be severe enough to cause arousal and ultimately produce chronic sleep deprivation.

Myoclonic jerks are often seen with diffuse CNS dysfunction of a variety of etiologies including acute intoxications, Alzheimer's disease, and viral encephalitis. They are a particularly common finding in Jakob-Creutzfeldt disease. All of those conditions may be manifested by behavior change. Also, in myoclonic epilepsy and occasionally in idiopathic epilepsy, individuals may experience numerous and even temporarily disabling myoclonic jerks after awakening in the morning. This peculiar symptom and the resulting limitation of activity may mistakenly be considered "psychological" in origin.

Hemiballismus refers to sudden, particularly violent movements of half of the body. It is an unusual symptom, and the pathology almost always includes a lesion in the subthalamic nucleus. The symptom usually develops rapidly, improves with time, and most commonly is the result of a vascular lesion.

Tremor refers to an oscillation of the neck, jaw, tongue, limbs, or trunk produced by alternating contractions of opposing muscles. It may be described as coarse or fine depending on its amplitude. It is convenient clinically to classify tremor by its relationship to movement. Tremor can occur at rest (resting tremor), with sustained posture of the limbs (postural tremor), and with voluntary movements (intention tremor). There is also a normal or physiologic tremor of small amplitude and high frequency that is present whenever muscles are actively contracting.

Tremor at rest most commonly occurs in parkinsonism, but may be seen with essential tremor and anxiety. Postural tremor is common with essential tremor, thyrotoxicosis, and lithium treatment. Sustained postures may also induce or exacerbate the tremor of parkinsonism. Intention tremor is commonly seen with disease of the cerebellum and with phenytoin toxicity.

Two other patterns worth noting are the wing-beating tremor of Wilson's disease (see the later discussion) and asterixis. Asterixis is a sudden and irregular flexion and extension of the wrist seen when this joint is maintained in a hyperextended posture. It may occur in a variety of intoxications and metabolic disorders, especially hepatic failure and uremia.

Neurobehavioral syndromes

This section will review syndromes in which abnormal movements and disordered behavior are often associated.

Huntington's chorea. Huntington's chorea is an autosomally dominant inherited disorder with onset usually in the fourth and fifth decades. It is characterized by progressive chorea and intellectual deterioration. With a knowledge of the family history, the diagnosis is straightforward. However, the family history is often hidden or poorly appreciated, and there is great variability in the presenting symptoms and rate of progression.

Intellectual impairment, impulsive or aggressive behavior, or frank psychosis may be the presenting phenomenon. Chorea may involve any group of muscles, but the trunk and proximal musculature are most commonly affected. As the disease progresses, twisting and lordotic movements of the trunk (especially when walking), associated with more intense arm and leg movements, give the individual a dancing, prancing gait that is characteristic of the disorder.

The chorea as well as the behavior disorder may be improved with neuroleptics, but the progress of the disease is not altered by any treatment. In the end stage choreatic movements often diminish, and a rigid akinetic state may develop. At this stage seizure phenomena are not uncommon, probably reflecting cortical involvement. An unusual form of Huntington's chorea begins in childhood with proximal muscle rigidity and seizures (Westphal variant) (10).

At postmortem examination the brain is atrophic, with the cerebral cortex and caudate nuclei primarily affected. In advanced cases the striatum may be almost devoid of neurons, with only reactive gliosis seen. Postmortem examinations have shown a relatively selective decrease in the peptide neurotransmitter gamma aminobutyric acid (GABA) as well as in its synthesizing enzyme, glutamic acid decarboxylase (GAD). There is also a decline in choline acetyltransferase, an acetylcholine-synthesizing enzyme. This finding suggests that early in the disease specific neurotransmitter defects may disrupt the integrated output of the extrapyramidal system (11).

Wilson's disease. Hepatolenticular degeneration—Wilson's disease—is an autosomal recessive inherited disease with signs and symptoms of cirrhosis of the liver and CNS dysfunction. Pathological changes in the nervous system are most prominent in the basal ganglia but may be seen in the cortex, cerebellum, and elsewhere.

Wilson's disease is caused by a deficit in copper metabolism. The precise pathophysiology is unknown, but ultimately copper accumulates in the kidney, liver, brain, and cornea (manifested as Kayser-Fleischer rings). Diagnosis is usually confirmed by a decreased serum ceruloplasmin, decreased copper level in the blood, increased copper excretion in the urine, and increased copper in specimens of liver obtained through percutaneous biopsy.

Symptoms usually appear in the second and third decades. On occasion evidence of liver disease may precede neurologic dysfunction (12). Basal ganglia dysfunction predominates, with tremor, rigidity, and dystonic posturing. Tremor may be of any type, but the most common is a bizarre "wing-beating tremor" of the upper limbs that usually appears when the arms are raised. Behavioral symptoms may precede or overshadow other symptoms early in the disease and may mimic affective illness or frank psychosis.

If the disease is untreated, the patient lives an average of four to six years from the time of diagnosis. Treatment can be very successful; it consists of a copper-poor diet and penicillamine, a chelating agent that increases urinary excre-

tion of copper (13).

Parkinson's disease. The parkinsonian syndrome ("parkinsonism") is a symptom complex characterized by varying degrees of tremor, rigidity, bradykinesia, and poor postural reflexes. It is separable into two clinical entities: primary or Parkinson's disease and second-

---

When dealing with tardive dyskinesia, the clinician should ask if the movements are truly tardive dyskinesia, and if the patient needs to remain on neuroleptic agents.

---

ary or symptomatic parkinsonism (14). The latter syndrome may have many different etiologies including cerebrovascular disease, Alzheimer's changes, encephalitis, and the use of neuroleptic agents (see parkinsonism below). Parkinson's disease per se is a neurodegeneration selectively involving the dopaminergic cells of the substantia nigra; its cause is unknown.

Several behavioral issues should be mentioned. They include the relationship of Parkinson's disease to dementia, its relationship to depression, and the psychological and behavioral side effects of dopaminergic and anticholinergic drugs used in its treatment.

● Parkinson's and dementia. Change in intellectual function with Parkinson's disease has been reported, but the issue is far from clear (15). First, Parkinson's disease is commonly a disorder of advancing age, a time when other conditions causing dementia are not infrequent. Second, parkinsonism may result from a variety of pathophysiologic processes. Thus parkinsonism may be secondary to a more diffuse disease of the brain (for example, Alzheimer's changes or cerebrovascular disease), though basal ganglia symptoms may predominate for many years.

Third, the intrinsic or idiopathic degeneration of the nigrostriatal tract may exist as one component of a broader syndrome. Thus in Shy-Drager syndrome, where the main clinical features are autonomic dysfunction (particularly orthostatic hypotension), patients quite frequently have parkinsonian symptoms, particularly bradykinesia and rigidity. Postmortem studies of these patients show degeneration in the caudate nucleus, substantia nigra, locus ceruleus, vagus nucleus, and ventral and lateral horns of the spinal cord.

Thus the incidence of dementia with Parkinson's disease will depend on how carefully we distinguish between normal and secondary parkinsonism. One statement can be made clearly. The large majority of patients with longstanding classic Parkinson's disease do not suffer from functionally significant or limiting intellectual deficits. The development of intellectual impairment should always lead the clinician to consider concurrent conditions such as affective disorder, subdural hematoma, and drug effect.

● Parkinson's and depression. The diagnosis of depression in the Parkinson's patient may be difficult. These patients have many of the features that physicians rely on to establish the diagnosis of major affective illness. They characteristically have an expressionless, masklike facies, difficulty sleeping, concerns about their loss of functional capacity, vague somatic complaints, and a significant degree of social withdrawal because they are unable to keep up with their peers or family obligations or are embarrassed by their appearance.

The problems confronting the consultant who evaluates an individual patient have also complicated studies of larger patient populations. It is difficult to devise an "objective" rating scale that does not depend on the above signs and symptoms. Such well-developed scales as Beck's (16) are heavily weighted toward somatic complaints. Also, studies have tended to compare persons who have Parkinson's disease with normal controls rather than with other groups of patients with chronic and partially disabling illness. Perhaps the most reliable strategy is for the treating physician to watch carefully for changes in mood that seem out of proportion to recent changes in neurologic function.

The use of antidepressant treatment in Parkinson's disease may be complicated. Tricyclic antidepressants may exacerbate the anticholinergic side effects of drugs such as trihexyphenidyl and benztropine and worsen the orthostatic hypotension produced by L-dopa, Sinemet, or bromocriptine. MAO inhibitors have been avoided because of the possibility of inducing hypertensive crisis in patients treated with L-dopa.

In recent years a centrally acting MAO-B inhibitor has been used to treat Parkinson's disease. Though still experimental, such selective agents may prove useful for both Parkinson's disease and affective disorder. The use of electroconvulsive therapy (ECT) in Parkinson's disease remains to be clarified. Certainly in the past patients with parkinsonian symptoms were reported to deteriorate with ECT. Some recent studies have been more positive.

• Psychological side effects. Antiparkinsonian drugs produce a variety of psychiatric and behavioral side effects. Hallucinations and delusions as well as persistent suspiciousness and paranoid ideation may be seen with L-dopa and dopaminergic agonists as well as with the anticholinergic drugs. Anticholinergics can also produce a relatively selective deterioration of memory. Regardless of the contributing factors of morbid personality and subclinical neurologic dysfunction, these behavioral side effects usually disappear with reduction or discontinuation of specific medications (17).

Drug-induced dyskinesias
Antipsychotic drugs cause a variety of extrapyramidal syndromes. The discussion that follows will briefly review drug-induced parkinson-

ism, acute dystonia, akathisia, and the "rabbit syndrome" (18) as well as amphetamine-induced dyskinesias, and then focus on tardive dyskinesia.

Parkinsonism is usually observed between the first and fourth weeks of treatment with antipsychotic agents. Rigidity, bradykinesia, and gait disorder are more common than tremor. All patients do not necessarily exhibit the full symptom complex, but mild symptoms such as diminished facial expressiveness, lack of blinking, and some loss of coordination are very common.

Evidence from animal experiments suggests a genetically determined intraspecies variability in the density of dopamine receptors in the corpus striatum; indeed, the variability in the development of parkinsonian symptoms may reflect a variability in the "reserve capacity" of the basal ganglia as well as in the total dosage necessary to control psychotic symptoms. Drug-induced parkinsonism tends to improve when the neuroleptic agent is reduced or discontinued and can be treated with anticholinergic drugs.

The *acute dystonic reactions* present as slow movements or sustained postures of the tongue, face, eyes, neck, or trunk. They occur early in neuroleptic use, usually within the first week, and are more common with the more potent neuroleptics such as piperazine phenothiazines, thioxanthenes, and butyrophenones.

The dystonias may be mistaken for psychogenic symptoms or seizures. They usually remit very rapidly with parenteral agents such as benztropine or diphenhydramine; these drugs constitute a diagnostic test as well as therapy. When the etiology of the movement disorder is at all unclear, a placebo can be administered first. The dystonic reactions may persist for a considerable period of time following a neuroleptic dose, and several successive doses of antiparkinson medication may be necessary.

Akathisia refers to a restlessness with frequent or constant motor

activity usually accompanied by a vague, unpleasant sense of discomfort. It is usually observed within the first few months of treatment with neuroleptics. This symptom may respond incompletely to sedatives or anticholinergics and may persist until the neuroleptic agent is discontinued.

The *"rabbit syndrome"* is a tremor of the lips that appears late in treatment; thus initially it may be mistaken for tardive dyskinesia. However, its therapeutic response to anticholinergic drugs distinguishes it from tardive dyskinesia.

Dyskinesias resulting from the use of amphetamines and other stimulants (19). Amphetamines may produce a paranoid psychosis resembling schizophrenia as well as a manic but not necessarily psychotic syndrome characterized by racing thoughts, pressured speech, euphoria, and grandiosity. Abnormal movements may include bruxism, a tendency to touch and pick at parts of the body, and stereotyped, compulsive motor behavior or automatisms. With chronic amphetamine use the patient may appear to have a progressive syndrome. The relative absence of confusion and disorientation may initially reduce the physician's suspicion that he is dealing with a toxic psychosis. Treatment here would consist of withdrawal of the drug and management of behavior with neuroleptics. Movement disorder can also occur in children with minimal brain dysfunction who are treated with amphetamines and methylphenidate.

Tardive dyskinesia is the most variable and potentially confusing of the movement disorders seen with antipsychotic drugs. Though it may resolve after a period of time when the drug is discontinued, it is not necessarily reversible. The most common abnormal movements are choreoathetosis of the lips, face, and tongue, but chorea of the limbs, shoulders, and pelvis as well as dystonic postures of the neck and trunk are also seen. These movements are more common in older patients. They usually appear after months or years of neuroleptic use and often emerge when dosage is being reduced. They can often be suppressed by again increasing the neuroleptic dose.

It is not yet clear whether continued use of antipsychotic agents by patients who have developed tardive dyskinesia leads to a worsening and ultimate prolongation of their movement disorder. Current practice favors discontinuing antipsychotic medication if at all possible (20).

Various data support the view that tardive dyskinesia results from dopaminergic overactivity. They include the evidence that tardive dyskinesia becomes worse with the administration of L-dopa or a dopaminergic agonist such as bromocriptine, and that neuroleptics suppress tardive dyskinesia.

The actual mechanism of dopaminergic overactivity is not clear. Several hypotheses have been considered. One is that prolonged dopamine receptor blockade may produce increased receptor binding at the postsynaptic membrane—that is, a CNS parallel to the increase in receptor sites with denervation in the peripheral nervous system. The proliferation of the postsynaptic dopamine receptor is well demonstrated in laboratory animals treated with neuroleptic agents. Other possible mechanisms include increased dopamine release, which may occur because of a blockade of presynaptic, inhibitory autoreceptors on the dopaminergic cell (the existence of these receptors and their ability to reduce cell firing is well documented) or because of the failure of a negative feedback loop from the striatum to the substantia nigra (21).

Approaches to the treatment of tardive dyskinesia have involved trials of numerous drugs with inconsistent success. The trials have included low doses of L-dopa, apomorphine, and bromocriptine in an attempt to selectively stimulate the dopamine autoreceptor and thus reduce the firing of the dopaminergic cell; the use of further doses of neuroleptics to block the postsynaptic receptor and reduce the

effect of either increased dopamine release or increased receptor sensitivity; and efforts to increase the "central cholinergic tone" through the use of acetylcholine precursors such as choline or lecithin or the use of direct cholinergic agonists such as physostigmine.

The variety of therapeutic attempts bears witness to the lack of a satisfactory treatment. In confronting tardive dyskinesia the clinician must consider two questions. First, are the observed movements truly tardive dyskinesia? The mannerisms that occur with schizophrenia and the senile chorea seen in the elderly may be clinically indistinguishable from tardive dyskinesia. Also, neurologic disease may present first with behavior change, leading to the use of neuroleptic agents. The later development of abnormal movements may then reflect the underlying disease process rather than a response to medication. Second, does the patient need to remain on neuroleptic agents? When was the last attempt to reduce or discontinue medication? At the present time, we must assume that the continued use of neuroleptic agents can lead to a progressively more severe or permanent movement disorder.

The problem of tardive dyskinesia highlights the issue of the co-occurrence of disorders of behavior and disorders of movement. Abnormal movements may be a psychiatric symptom, a neurologic symptom of an illness that may also produce abnormal behavior, and/or a result of therapy. It is often a challenge for both the neurologist and the psychiatrist to distinguish cause and effect.

References

1. Calne DB: Developments in the pharmacology and therapeutics of parkinsonism. Annals of Neurology 1:111–119, 1977
2. Crothers B, Paine RS: The Natural History of Cerebral Palsy. Cambridge, Mass, Harvard University Press, 1959
3. Plaitakis A: The olivopontocerebellar atrophies. Seminars in Neurology 2:334–340, 1982
4. Shapiro AK, Shapiro E: Tourette syndrome: clinical aspects, treatment, and etiology. Seminars in Neurology 2:373–385, 1982
5. Duvoisin RC: Chorea. Seminars in Neurology 2:351–358, 1982
6. Marsden CD: Dystonia: the spectrum of the disease, in The Basal Ganglia. Edited by Yahr MD. New York, Raven, 1976
7. Eldridge R: The torsion dystonias: literature review and genetic and clinical studies. Neurology 20:1–78, 1970
8. Sheehy MP, Marsden CD: Writers' cramp: a focal dystonia. Brain 105 (pt 3):461–480, 1982
9. Fahn S: Treatment of dystonia with high-dosage anticholinergic medication. Neurology 29:605–612, 1979
10. Byers RK, Gilles FH, Fong C: Huntington's disease in children. Neurology 23:561–569, 1973
11. Bird ED: Chemical pathology of Huntington's disease. Annual Review of Pharmacology and Toxicology 20:533–551, 1980
12. Slovis TL, Dubois RS, Rogerson D, et al: The varied manifestations of Wilson's disease. Journal of Pediatrics 78:578–584, 1971
13. Scheinberg IH, Sternlieb I: Wilson's disease, in Biology of Brain Dysfunction, vol 3. Edited by Gaull GE. New York, Raven, 1975
14. Yahr MD: The parkinsonian syndrome, in A Textbook of Neurology, 6th ed. Edited by Merritt HH. Philadelphia, Lea & Febiger, 1979
15. Bowen FP, Brady EM, Yahr MD: Short and long range studies of memory, intelligence, and perception in Parkinson patients treated with levodopa, in Parkinson's Disease: Rigidity, Akinesia, Behavior, vol 2. Edited by Siegfried J. Bern, Hans Hoeber, 1972
16. Beck AT: Depression. Philadelphia, University of Pennsylvania Press, 1970
17. Yahr MD, Korczyn A: Psychiatric side-effects of antiparkinson drugs, in Geriatric Psychopharmacology. Edited by Nandy K. New York, Elsevier/North-Holland, 1979
18. Baldessarini RJ: Drugs and the treatment of psychiatric disorders, in the Pharmacological Basis of Therapeutics, 6th ed. Edited by Gilman AG, Goodman LS, Gilman A. New York, Macmillan, 1980
19. Randrop A, Munkuad I: Biochemical, anatomical, and psychological investigations of stereotyped behavior induced by amphetamines, in International Symposium on Amphetamines and Related Compounds. Edited by Costa E, Garattini S. New York, Raven, 1970
20. Klawans HL, Goetz CG, Perlik S: Tardive dyskinesia: review and update. American Journal of Psychiatry 137:900–908, 1980
21. Baldessarini RJ, Tarsy D: Dopamine and the pathophysiology of dyskinesias induced by antipsychotic drugs. Annual Review of Neuroscience 3:23–41, 1980

Overcoming Resistance to Talking to Patients About Tardive Dyskinesia

Mark R. Munetz, M.D.

The American Psychiatric Association's task force report on tardive dyskinesia recommends that when a clinician wishes to prescribe a maintenance regimen of neuroleptic drugs, patients and families be advised of the risks and benefits so that a mutual decision can be made. However, there is significant resistance to talking to patients about tardive dyskinesia. The author reviews institutional, clinician, and patient sources of this resistance and describes ways that obstacles to obtaining informed consent can be overcome. He concludes that with strong institutional support, clinicians functioning as a team can learn to view patient education and involvement in decision-making as an integral part of treatment.

The American Psychiatric Association's task force report on tardive dyskinesia contains guidelines for the avoidance of and management of tardive dyskinesia (1). Included is the suggestion that when clinicians recommend an ongoing course of neuroleptic medication, patients and families should be advised of the risks and benefits of neuroleptic drugs so that a mutual

Dr. Munetz is assistant professor of psychiatry at Western Psychiatric Institute and Clinic, University of Pittsburgh School of Medicine, 3811 O'Hara Street, Pittsburgh, Pennsylvania 15213. The author acknowledges the assistance of Loren H. Roth, M.D., and Catherine Scala, R.N., M.S.N.

decision can be reached.

The outpatient schizophrenia clinic at the Western Psychiatric Institute and Clinic adopted the APA guidelines in 1983, including the policy of verbally obtaining informed consent for maintenance neuroleptic therapy. This policy decision was based partly on a study over several years of the process of obtaining consent from tardive dyskinesia patients (2,3).

It has been apparent in our clinic that even though we have devoted a great deal of attention to the problem of tardive dyskinesia, there remains significant resistance to compliance with the informed consent guidelines. Discussions with clinicians throughout the country suggest that this resistance is widespread. Although the APA guidelines, published in 1979, have been receiving increasing publicity (4), they have yet to be universally adopted.

The purpose of this paper is to review the sources of resistance to obtaining informed consent for neuroleptic drugs. Institutional, therapist, and patient barriers will be discussed, along with suggested ways in which these obstacles can be overcome.

Institutional resistance

In a few states such as California and New Jersey judicial decisions have mandated that informed consent be obtained for the administration of neuroleptic drugs (5,6). But otherwise there has been little impetus until recently for institutions to develop policies to obtain informed consent for the routine administration of neuroleptics. Although the interest in providing optimal clinical care as well as a

fear of lawsuits might stimulate an institution to establish an informed consent standard, paradoxically these same concerns have provided the rationale for *not* developing an informed consent policy. It has been argued, for example, that good clinical care dictates that patients not be frightened, and thus driven out of treatment, by information about potential side effects. Similarly it has been argued that lawsuits are more likely to occur if clinicians now begin telling patients about the risks of neuroleptic treatment when in fact the decision to use neuroleptics was made years earlier, often in a different treatment setting.

However, data from our own study and ongoing clinical experience suggest that patients do not respond to information about tardive dyskinesia with tremendous anxiety or by fleeing treatment in large numbers (2,3). While the fear of lawsuits may be realistic, the longer an agency waits to begin informing its patients about the risk of tardive dyskinesia, the greater its vulnerability to charges of negligence. As the professional community and the general public become more informed about tardive dyskinesia (4), institutional silence becomes increasingly indefensible.

Once an agency decides on the need for an informed consent policy, it must decide whether to follow APA's suggestion of holding an informal discussion and documenting it (1) or using a written consent form, as others have suggested (7,8). Written consent forms may appeal to institutions because they are readily available, provide concrete evidence that consent has been obtained, and can be incorporated into routine paperwork with minimal expenditure of clinician time. Our experience suggests, however, that the use of written consent forms does not increase patient knowledge any more than informal discussion does and may foster the view of consent as a one-time process (2,3). Thus although written consent is easy to obtain, it may be clinically unhelpful and carry little legal weight (9,10).

Ideally, informed consent should be considered an ongoing process that is an integral part of treatment in such a way that patients and families can be actively involved in medical decision-making. Viewed in this way, informed consent requires a significant commitment of clinician time. Which clinicians should devote time to this form of patient education?

While clearly the physician is ultimately responsible for prescribing neuroleptics, in a clinic setting a nonphysician primary therapist commonly spends the most time directly with patients. In addition, a medication nurse may provide care to patients, especially those receiving injectable drugs.

If an agency does not have clear guidelines about who is responsible for information disclosure, two types of problems may result. The first is the buck-passing phenomenon. The physician rationalizes that although he is prescribing the medication, it is more appropriate for the primary therapist, who knows the patient best, to discuss consent issues. Conversely, the therapist reasons that the physician who prescribes the medication should be responsible for disclosing adequate information. The nurse who actually administers the medication believes that she is simply following the doctor's orders and is not authorized to discuss sensitive information. Thus no one provides the information.

The second problem occurs if the treating physician designates that only he may discuss the important medical issue of tardive dyskinesia. Other members of the

treatment team are strictly prohibited from discussing this issue with patients or families.

This situation is fraught with problems. Excluding from the education process the clinicians who see the patient most often decreases the likelihood that patients will learn over time what they need to know. If on the other hand the physician educates all members of the treatment team about the use of neuroleptic drugs for chronic mental illness so that in turn they can educate patients, the ideal of informed consent may be better realized.

In some situations, the physician takes control of information disclosure not to facilitate informed consent but on the grounds of therapeutic privilege, the concept that the physician can withhold information if he believes that disclosing it will be harmful to the patient (11). Specifically, physicians sometimes withhold information about tardive dyskinesia because they believe that the patient will refuse to continue taking the medication. However, therapeutic privilege cannot be invoked simply because the physician believes that disclosure will result in treatment refusal; competent patients have the right to refuse treatment.

Therapists' resistance

Compounding institutional inertia is the resistance therapists themselves have to discussing tardive dyskinesia with patients. It is not surprising that therapists do not rush to tell all their patients about the long-term risks of neuroleptics. In the hope of maintaining a fragile working alliance, it is especially tempting to withhold information about tardive dyskinesia from hostile, paranoid, or very ambivalent, uninsightful patients. Some unremittingly paranoid patients do use knowledge about tardive dyskinesia as one more piece of evidence that the physician is not to be trusted and that medication should be avoided. However, in our experience those patients generally have not complied with medication regimens long before

they were told about tardive dyskinesia.

More commonly, we find that patients only tenuously involved in a treatment alliance respond positively to their therapists' attempts to provide information to help them participate actively in treatment decision-making. As Lion (12) has suggested, display of openness works both in building trust and in negating perceived struggles for control. The process transcends any alarming effect of the disclosed information itself.

But even for those who embrace the concept of collaborative, informed decision-making, it remains especially difficult to talk to patients about tardive dyskinesia. Two aspects of tardive dyskinesia and neuroleptic treatment may contribute to this difficulty. First, unlike many potentially serious side effects, tardive dyskinesia is more than a theoretical risk. Prevalence with long-term neuroleptic treatment is conservatively estimated at 10 to 20 percent (1), and a recent study reports an incidence of more than 3 percent per year (13). While severe, irreversible tardive dyskinesia is rare, clinicians painfully recognize that neuroleptics not infrequently do harm patients.

Second, in talking to patients about tardive dyskinesia, clinicians must confront their own beliefs about the value of neuroleptic drugs. Research data overwhelmingly support the effectiveness of neuroleptics in both acute and prophylactic treatment of many schizophrenic patients (14), but there remains a significant population who, despite neuroleptic treatment, have chronic active psychotic symptoms or predominantly negative or defect-state symptoms. These patients remain highly dysfunctional. Their poor response raises vital and legitimate questions about the benefits of ongoing neuroleptic treatment. It is difficult for a therapist to face the possibility that neuroleptics have been prescribed for a patient for years without clear evidence of benefit. It is psychologically easier not to raise the question and simply continue prescribing the drugs.

Thus in initiating discussion with patients about tardive dyskinesia, therapists are forced to face the limitations and the hazards of the only effective treatment for schizophrenia they know.

Patient barriers

Early in their treatment, schizophrenic patients may be too disorganized to listen to, understand, or process the information they need to arrive at a rational treatment decision. The disorganized paranoid patient who denies being ill at all is not likely to agree to the need for neuroleptic medication under any circumstance.

Stable, more insightful patients may still present obstacles to collaborative decision-making. Some patients either do not want to be informed about medication or do not wish to make treatment decisions; they prefer to leave the decisions up to the doctor. Such a waiver of rights is totally acceptable under the doctrine of informed consent (11).

Also common but more problematic are patients who seem interested in being active decision-makers but, despite therapists' intensive efforts to educate them, do not absorb or retain the information therapists consider necessary for making an informed decision (2). While it has been argued that such patients are incompetent (15), they often clearly are not. They are rarely legally incompetent (that is, they have not been adjudicated as such by a court), and in fact they function as independent decision-makers in their daily lives.

Also related to the question of patient competence is the finding that approximately half of the patients who have tardive dyskinesia deny awareness of their involuntary movements (8,16). The problem is how patients can consider the risks of a side effect they do not believe exists (8).

Involving family members in the consent process may allay some of the clinician's concern that the medication decision is made by a de facto incompetent patient. However, many older chronic mental patients do not have family members available. Moreover, including family members in decision-making may not always be appropriate (17). Sometimes an adult schizophrenic patient wishes to

---

More problematic are patients who, despite their interest in decision-making, do not absorb or retain the information necessary for making an informed decision.

---

make an independent decision about a course of action to which the family objects. For example, relatives of a patient with tardive dyskinesia may be very disturbed by his involuntary movements and request discontinuation of neuroleptics. The patient, on the other hand, may be undisturbed by the movements but tremendously fearful of a psychotic relapse. The physician must try to help patient and family balance the Scylla of recurrent psychosis with the Charybdis of persistent dyskinesia, but ultimately the legally competent patient has the right to make the final decision about continuing medication.

Overcoming the obstacles

Ideally, informed consent should be viewed as an ongoing process involving all members of the treatment team in such a way that patient education becomes an integral part of routine clinical practice. Before therapists can begin to translate this ideal into practice, however, there must be strong, clear institutional support for a policy of obtaining meaningful informed consent for neuroleptic drugs. Such institutional support is likely to increase as the APA guidelines become established by

litigation as a standard for care (4) and as media attention to tardive dyskinesia increases.

As noted, however, even an institutional mandate does not make it easy for clinicians to discuss very specific, sensitive information with schizophrenic patients. The fear of harming patients by causing them to discontinue medication remains the greatest source of inhibition. Therapists can overcome this anxiety by the progressive desensitization that occurs when they begin discussing tardive dyskinesia with patients and get positive results. In our experience, the more a clinician talks to patients about these issues, the easier it becomes.

When and how to talk to patients

The informed consent process should begin as soon as it is clinically feasible. The earlier the first discussion about neuroleptic medication takes place, the easier more detailed discussions become in the future. Although tardive dyskinesia generally does not occur until after several years of neuroleptic exposure, it sometimes occurs sooner, and the presumed time lag does not justify delaying disclosure of information (18).

The determination of when to initiate discussion of neuroleptics must be based on the therapist's clinical judgment of when the patient is able to begin to understand the information necessary to weigh the risks and benefits. For highly disturbed, acutely psychotic patients, it may be necessary to wait for several days or weeks after the institution of neuroleptics. For less severely disturbed patients, the informed consent process should begin before the administration of drugs (18).

If the patient agrees to it, it is appropriate to include relatives in the discussions about medication. If the clinician believes the patient is not able to make a meaningful decision about treatment, then the clinician should try to obtain proxy consent from friends, relatives, or institutional committees (18).

Although we do not advocate

the use of written consent forms, there are other instruments that may facilitate the informed consent process. They include the Abnormal Involuntary Movement Scale (AIMS) examination (19), a patient questionnaire or postdisclosure test (2,20), medication information booklets, and medication groups.

The administration of a screening test like the AIMS examination is recommended every three to six months to help assess the presence and severity of involuntary movements (1). Routine, periodic AIMS examinations provide a natural introduction to routine, periodic discussions with patients about tardive dyskinesia.

We have learned that therapists find some sort of structure helpful in discussing the risks and benefits of neuroleptic drugs with patients. Consent forms seem inadequate for this purpose, but the administration of a questionnaire or test to patients both before and, especially, after discussions about tardive dyskinesia provides a useful structure (2). The questionnaire not only can remind the therapist of issues that should be covered but can also be used to help gauge patient knowledge before and after each discussion. Thus a questionnaire can be both a teaching instrument and an assessment instrument for the patient and clinician.

The American Medical Association has developed patient medication instruction sheets that contain basic information about the uses and side effects of specific medications, including neuroleptics. More detailed booklets can be used to help educate patients or their families and to stimulate questions for further discussion.

Medication groups are another means of facilitating discussion about tardive dyskinesia. In a group setting patients can complement the work of the therapist and educate each other. Statements from peers frequently carry more weight than those from professionals, and in our experience patients frequently get to the core of other patients' resistance. Furthermore,

patients suffering from tardive dyskinesia not only graphically demonstrate the disorder but may be able to discuss their view of the burden of tardive dyskinesia compared with the burden of recurrent psychosis.

What to say to patients

There is no rote discussion adequate for every patient, but we can outline some general principles that may help alleviate therapists' anxiety about talking to patients about tardive dyskinesia.

To begin with, discussion should be informal. A conversational style using the simplest possible language will be far more effective than a scientific discourse. The tone should be supportive but frank.

The therapist should give the patient his view of the nature of his psychiatric illness, describe the indications for maintenance neuroleptics, and discuss the availability or unavailability of alternative treatments. Patients need to be told the risks of continuing treatment, specifically tardive dyskinesia. It is important for patients to know that tardive dyskinesia generally is the result of long-term neuroleptic drug use and is potentially irreversible. They should also understand that the likelihood of reversibility may be increased with early detection.

Our understanding of tardive dyskinesia is changing, and a great deal about the disorder remains unknown. Thus we cannot present "all the facts" to our patients. What we must share with them, along with the established facts about the condition, is the uncertainty.

The therapist may want to convey his personal distress about the uncertainty surrounding tardive dyskinesia as well as about the lack of an effective treatment. The therapist then may explain the need for periodic examinations, to enlist the patient's help in early detection of involuntary movements and to allow for rapid intervention while the movements are still reversible. In our experience patients are reassured to know that therapists are

actively looking for evidence of this dreaded side effect.

It is reassuring to both patient and therapist if the responsibility for weighing the risks and benefits of neuroleptic drugs is shared. Although the therapist is obligated to answer the question "What would you do if you were in my shoes?"—that is, to give a professional recommendation (21)—the patient has the right to make the final treatment decision.

The amount of information presented should vary according to the patient's clinical status, interest, and intellect. It is important to emphasize that all information need not be presented in a single session. There is always the opportunity for subsequent repetition and elaboration. Telling the patient in one session that you plan to say more in the next session can be a useful way for both the patient and the clinician to be prepared for a more detailed discussion. The aim is that the patient gradually will become more knowledgeable about his treatment and its side effects.

It is not clear that a patient needs to meet a minimum standard of knowledge to become a competent decision-maker (22). What patients do need to know is that neuroleptic treatment carries both risks and benefits, that they have the right to weigh the two and, if they wish, arrive at a decision to begin or continue medication. One hopes that such a decision is influenced by a considered professional recommendation, but the patient has the right to make the final decision. Knowing that one has a choice about one's pharmacotherapy and being free to make such a choice is probably the most important outcome of the informed consent process.

References

1. Tardive Dyskinesia: Report of the American Psychiatric Association Task Force on Late Neurological Effects of Antipsychotic Drugs. APA Task Force Report 18. Washington, DC, American Psychiatric Association, 1979

2. Munetz MR, Roth LH, Cornes CL: Tardive dyskinesia and informed consent: myths and realities. Bulletin of the American Academy of Psychiatry and the Law 10:77–88, 1982
3. Munetz MR, Roth LH: Informing patients about tardive dyskinesia. Archives of General Psychiatry (in press)
4. Herrington B: Tardive dyskinesia court cases underscore importance of APA report. Psychiatric News, Oct 7, 1983
5. Title 9, California Administrative Code, subchapter 4, article 5.5, section 851, 1980
6. Rennie v Klein, 476 F Supp 1294, 1309–10 (DNJ 1979)
7. Sovner R, DiMascio A, Berkowitz D, et al: Tardive dyskinesia and informed consent. Psychosomatics 19:172–177, 1978
8. DeVeaugh-Geiss J: Informed consent for neuroleptic therapy. American Journal of Psychiatry 136:959–962, 1979
9. Vaccarino JM: Consent, informed consent, and the consent form (edtl). New England Journal of Medicine 298:455, 1978
10. Slovenko R: On the legal aspects of tardive dyskinesia. Journal of Psychiatry and Law 7:295–331, 1979
11. Meisel A: The "exceptions" to informed consent: striking a balance between competing values in medical decision-making. Wisconsin Law Review 1979:413–488, 1979
12. Lion JR: The Art of Medicating Psychiatric Patients. Baltimore, Williams & Wilkins, 1978
13. Kane JM, Woerner M, Weinhold P, et al: Incidence of tardive dyskinesia: five-year data from a prospective study. Psychopharmacology Bulletin 20:39–40, 1984
14. Davis JM: Overview: maintenance therapy in psychiatry: I, schizophrenia. American Journal of Psychiatry 132:1237–1245, 1975
15. Grossman L, Summer F: A study of the capacity of schizophrenic patients to give informed consent. Hospital and Community Psychiatry 31:205–206, 1980
16. Alexopoulos GS: Lack of complaints in schizophrenics with tardive dyskinesia. Journal of Nervous and Mental Disease 167:125–127, 1979
17. Angell M: Respecting the autonomy of competent patients. New England Journal of Medicine 310:1115–1116, 1984
18. Roth LH: Question the experts. Journal of Clinical Psychopharmacology 3:207–208, 1983
19. Guy W: ECDEU Assessment Manual for Psychopharmacology, Revised 1976. Washington, DC, US Department of Health, Education, and Welfare, 1976
20. Miller R, Willner SH: The two-part consent form: a suggestion for promoting free and informed consent. New England Journal of Medicine 290:964–966, 1974
21. Ingelfinger FJ: Arrogance. New England Journal of Medicine 303:1507–1511, 1980
22. Appelbaum PS, Roth LH: Competency to consent to research: a psychiatric overview. Archives of General Psychiatry 39:951–958, 1982

Law & Psychiatry

Legal Liability for Tardive Dyskinesia

Robert M. Wettstein, M.D.
Paul S. Appelbaum, M.D.,
Editor

Probably few mental health professionals are unaware of or unaffected by the threat of malpractice litigation in daily clinical practice. Recent reports in the psychiatric literature reveal both increasing frequency and severity of claims filed by psychiatrists. In 1982 one of every 25 psychiatrists insured through the American Psychiatric Association malpractice program filed an insurance claim, at an average estimated cost, for 1983 claims, of $55,000 (1). While serious or fatal physical injuries including suicide account for much financial loss by the malpractice insurance program, claims for psychological and less severe physical injuries are also considerable.

Of derivative interest is the specter of malpractice litigation surrounding psychotropic drug reactions, particularly tardive dyskinesia and tardive dystonia. Now well recognized as a prevalent result of the use of neuroleptic drugs in psychiatric inpatients and outpatients, tardive dyskinesia and tardive dystonia command much

Dr. Wettstein is assistant professor of psychiatry at Western Psychiatric Institute and Clinic, 3811 O'Hara Street, Pittsburgh, Pennsylvania 15213. Dr. Appelbaum is A. F. Zeleznik professor of psychiatry and director of the law and psychiatry program at the University of Massachusetts Medical School in Worcester.

more serious respect and concern than just a few years earlier. Still, a great number of lawsuits for neuroleptic-induced movement disorders have yet to be filed; in fact, Slawson reported that such suits were infrequent (1). Two recent cases with sizable judgments against mental health professionals and medical care facilities, however, deserve comment.

In *Clites v. State of Iowa* (2), the parents of a mentally retarded patient at a state hospital–school brought action against the hospital for medical malpractice. The patient had first entered the state residential facility when he was 11. At age 18, he began receiving a variety of antipsychotic medications to manage his "aggressive behavior" under the auspices of several different physicians. Medication continued for five years before the patient was diagnosed as having tardive dyskinesia of the face and extremities.

After hearing expert testimony about the standard of care for such a patient, the trial court determined that medication had been inappropriately used for the convenience of the staff and not for the treatment of the patient, and that evidence of the severe aggression and self-destructiveness required to justify such use of major tranquilizers was lacking. The court also ruled that the patient was improperly monitored because "he was not regularly visited by a physician and physical exams had not been conducted for a three-year period"; the staff, without justification, ignored the known risks of uninterrupted use of major tranquilizers; the medical staff failed to react to the patient's symptoms of

tardive dyskinesia and alter the drug treatment program accordingly; and the attending physician, being unfamiliar with tardive dyskinesia, failed to obtain consultation. The court further stated that polypharmacy was not warranted by the patient's status and the particular drugs involved and that the patient's "parents were never informed of the potential side effects of the use, and prolonged use, of major tranquilizers, nor was consent to their use obtained," thus violating the "standard that requires some form of informed consent prior to the administration of major tranquilizers."

The trial court rejected the defendant's argument that the patient's parents implicitly consented to the treatment, since they were not informed of the risks attendant to the treatment program. The trial court ruled for the plaintiff and awarded $385,165 for future medical expenses and $375,000 for past and future pain and suffering. The district court's ruling was subsequently upheld in the Iowa Court of Appeals (3).

Faigenbaum v. Oakland Medical Center (4) concerns a 50-year-old woman who began to experience symptoms of tardive dyskinesia involving her face and limbs in 1976, after an undetermined number of years of antipsychotic drug treatment starting in 1964. The patient had been treated in the past as an outpatient and an inpatient for a recurrent depressive disorder but had also been diagnosed as suffering from a schizophrenic disorder.

In 1976 she admitted herself to a state psychiatric hospital for evaluation and treatment of her movement disorder and remained there for more than a year. During this time her movement disorder progressed to involve her face, neck, mouth, throat, extremities, and gait; she was referred for neurological evaluation at the adjacent state medical-surgical center. A neurologist employed by the medical center diagnosed Huntington's chorea, although the patient's family history was negative for the disease; the neurologist recommended that the patient be treated with antipsychotic medication.

During the patient's psychiatric hospitalization in 1976 and 1977 neuroleptics were prescribed by several treating psychiatrists who relied on the neurologist's diagnosis in preference to a diagnosis of tardive dyskinesia made by other consulting physicians. Her antipsychotic medication was later discontinued at the family's request, and the patient was discharged with a diagnosis of Huntington's chorea and hysterical neurosis, conversion type

Her family then obtained medical consultation elsewhere and a diagnosis of tardive dyskinesia was made. Suit was brought against the consulting neurologist, eight psychiatrists, two internists, the state psychiatric hospital, the state medical–surgical facility, and several manufacturers of antipsychotic medications. Causes of action against the physicians included negligent failure to consider tardive dyskinesia within a differential diagnosis, failure to obtain a drug or neurological history, and improper prescription of antipsychotic medication. The psychiatrists in particular were alleged to have acted improperly by relying exclusively on the consultant's diagnosis and report.

The plaintiff settled for $378,000 in damages against several defendants, including the neurologist, the three psychiatrists, and the two hospitals that had treated her before her state hospitalization. The trial court determined that governmental immunity for state psychiatric institutions and their employees shielded the state psychiatric hospital and three other psychiatrists from liability. The state medical–surgical facility was not immune from suit, and a $1 million jury verdict was obtained, plus $350,000 for costs and interest. Subsequent settlements totaling $100,000 from pharmaceutical manufacturers for inadequate warnings to physicians of the risks of tardive dyskinesia were also obtained. Damages were assessed for medical expenses, compensation for injuries, and pain and suffering, but not for lost wages or future earnings (5).

While such cases are disquieting, few psychiatrists should find reason to despair. It is probably premature to assess the general direction of case-law developments in this area, though more of such litigation can be anticipated. Further, while recent case law pertaining to the right to refuse treatment has exaggerated the risks of antipsychotic medication in comparison to its benefits (6), there is little indication of such a pervasive prejudice in the judicial system as a whole.

Litigation concerning tardive dyskinesia is grounded in two areas of malpractice—negligence in the diagnosis and treatment of major mental disorders and failure to obtain informed consent (7). Successful action under either theory presupposes a failure to meet a nationally derived standard of care in the practice of psychiatry, rather than the presence of an adverse consequence per se, which would occur in a strict liability model.

As long as negligence remains the legal standard for determining liability for physicians' services, the risk of liability is subject to intervention. Litigation should at least theoretically provide a healthy incentive to practitioners and institutions to ensure compliance with standard care, yet the typical development of tardive dyskinesia after treatment with antipsychotic medication over an extended period of time, prescribed by perhaps several physicians at different institutions, obfuscates such incentives. In such a situation often involving several treating and consulting physicians, a physician may find it easy to neglect his or her own responsibility to the patient. Nevertheless, all practitioners ultimately bear the financial, social, and emotional costs incurred by negligent physicians (8).

Thus physicians, agencies, and hospitals need appropriate written policies and procedures for the systematic monitoring of patients being treated with antipsychotic medication, whether or not tardive dyskinesia and tardive dystonia are present (9). Such policies could be included under existing guidelines with regard to the appropriate use and dosage of antipsychotic and antiparkinsonian medications, but would also address the need for periodic evaluation for tardive dyskinesia; the use of standardized dyskinesia-assessment instruments; the role of consulting neurologists in screening, diagnosis, and treatment of tardive dyskinesia; the availability of costly neurological diagnostic procedures (electroencephalogram or computerized tomography, for example); and the method of securing and periodically renewing a meaningful informed consent from the patient or his or her legal guardian both on the use of antipsychotic medication and the management of tardive dyskinesia. The formulation of such a policy demands a consensus among clinical (psychiatric and neurologic), administrative, legal, financial, and ethical agendas.

It has long been known, however, that "incidents don't sue, patients do"; that is, litigation is predicated on something more than even egregious medical error (10). Although there is no substitute for good clinical practice, we must not overlook the relevant relationships among the parties to the psychiatric transaction—the patient, patient's family or guardian, prescribing and consulting physicians, and institution. While we have just begun to understand the risk factors for the development of tardive dyskinesia, we know even less about the risk factors for its litigation.

References

1. Slawson PE: The clinical dimension of psychiatric malpractice. Psychiatric Annals 14:358–364, 1984
2. Clites v State of Iowa, Law No 46274, Iowa District Court, Pottawattamie County, Aug 7, 1980
3. Clites v State of Iowa, 322 NW2d 917, 1982
4. Faigenbaum v Oakland Medical Center, et al, Wayne County Circuit Court, No. 79-904–736, NM, July 27, 1982
(Continued on page 39)

Psychopharmacology

Training Hospital Clinicians to Diagnose Tardive Dyskinesia

Christopher K. Germer,
Ph.D.
Louisa Seraydarian, M.Ed.
John F. McBrearty, Ph.D.

Tardive dyskinesia is a major concern because it is an iatrogenic disorder, appears to be increasingly prevalent (1), and is irreversible in many cases (2). The disorder is a gradually appearing extrapyramidal side effect of neuroleptic medication characterized by a wide variety of involuntary movements, including lip smacking, chewing, sucking, tongue thrusting, and jaw movements. Occasionally tardive dyskinesia also includes flapping and writhing (choreiform) movements of the extremities, dystonic posturing of the neck and trunk, and respiration difficulties.

Tardive dyskinesia is commonly found in 15 to 25 percent of patients being treated with neuroleptics (1,3); in up to 55 percent of the cases it develops within three years of continuous exposure to drugs (3). The disorder is persistent in at least one-third of all cases (4–6). Evidence suggests that tardive dyskinesia may remit, partially or fully, if it is diagnosed early

Dr. Germer is a research coordinator and Ms. Seraydarian and Dr. McBrearty are co-directors at the program evaluation department, Haverford State Hospital, 3500 Darby Road, Haverford, Pennsylvania 19041. Address correspondence to Dr. McBrearty. The authors thank John K. Fong, D.O., Theodore Barry, M.D., and Florence Pecha, R.N., for their advice and support throughout the project, and the physicians and nurses who performed the patient examinations.

and neuroleptics are discontinued or dosages are reduced.

There is unfortunately no laboratory test to diagnose tardive dyskinesia, and there is a lack of satisfactory treatment (8). Under these circumstances, the busy clinician may be inclined to overlook the disorder in its initial, reversible stages. This omission may have serious consequences in a psychiatric hospital such as ours, in which 88 percent of all patients receive neuroleptics regularly or on an as-needed basis.

Although psychiatrists are becoming aware of tardive dyskinesia through a spate of articles in recent years, there is relatively little in the literature regarding practical identification and quantification of the disorder by hospital clinicians. Assessment of tardive dyskinesia has typically been carried out by a few specially trained researchers.

To establish the prevalence of movement disorders, particularly tardive dyskinesia, the program evaluation department at Haverford State Hospital developed a tardive dyskinesia prevalence survey and a program to train staff members to recognize subtle movement disorders that ordinarily remain undetected. The survey and training program consist of five phases: diagnostic training, patient evaluation, chart review, symptom management, and patient reevaluation.

This paper presents the training program only, which involves active, yet limited, participation by psychiatric staff, and which may be adapted for use in any hospital. Inquiries regarding the survey, which is being processed and the findings prepared for publication, should be addressed to the second author (LS).

Diagnostic training

The Abnormal Involuntary Movement Scale (AIMS), a widely used assessment instrument developed by the psychopharmacology research branch of the National Institute of Mental Health (NIMH) (9), was selected for the physical measurement and clinical quantification of tardive dyskinesia. It has good interrater and test/retest reliability (10,11), and allows staff to easily detect abnormal movements that go unrecognized during routine interaction with patients.

To provide a common basis for defining cases of tardive dyskinesia, Schooler and Kane (12) developed formal diagnostic criteria for AIMS. The criteria for probable tardive dyskinesia are a history of at least three months of continuous exposure to neuroleptics; the presence of at least moderate abnormal involuntary movements in one or more body areas or at least mild movements in two or more body areas; and the absence of other conditions that might produce involuntary movements. Patient reexamination is necessary to determine if the symptoms are transient or persistent.

Four psychiatrists at Haverford State Hospital were pretrained by the program coordinator to act as AIMS instructors. They in turn instructed groups of four to eight volunteers to reliably score patients on AIMS. Fifteen psychiatrists, 15 registered nurses, and nine hospital admission physicians volunteered to participate in the three-hour training session.

The training sessions used a videotape provided by the psychopharmacology research branch of NIMH. Participants viewed patients with tardive dyskinesia, made AIMS ratings of the patients, and then compared their ratings to those on the videotape. Inconsistent scoring was discussed by the group. Instructors then discussed the differential diagnosis of movement disorders using the excellent review articles by Granacher (13) and the American Psychiatric Association task force on tardive dyskinesia (14). We recommend the videotape and review articles to those who wish to develop similar training programs.

The participants then made independent AIMS ratings of two videotaped tardive dyskinesia patients from Haverford Hospital. The interrater reliability alpha coefficient of 39 ratings of these two patients was very high (.97).

A few modifications suggested by Smith and associates (10,15,16) were instituted in the examination procedure used with the two Haverford patients. The patients were asked to remove their shoes so that better observations of toe movements could be made, and they remained in the examination room during the ratings so symptoms could be reevaluated if necessary. Scoring of severity did not depend on whether an abnormal movement increased when it was activated by movement in another body area, although activated movements were noted on the AIMS form.

Patients were also asked whether they noticed abnormal movements in themselves or in other patients. Previous research suggests that only one-third of patients are aware of their tardive dyskinesia (16). Since consent is received from most patients before the examination, some patients tend to conceal movements from the examiner by folding their legs or clenching their fists. Not being aware of one's own abnormal movements and yet seeing such movements in others presumably reflects conscious control of symptoms.

The AIMS raters were given a supplementary form, the other movement disorders checklist, to complete along with AIMS. We designed the checklist to facilitate differential diagnosis of tardive dyskinesia and abnormal movements related to parkinsonism, dystonia, akathisia, tics, and mannerisms. (The checklist is also available from the second author.)

Tardive dyskinesia is indistinguishable from some stereotypic movement disorders of schizophrenia, spontaneous oral dyskinesias in the elderly, and oral dyskinesias related to problems with teeth or dentures (12). Dental problems are noted on the AIMS form, and it is helpful to remove the patient's dentures before examination. Movements similar to those of tardive dyskinesia but unrelated to neuroleptic medication may be found in 25 percent of patients treated with neuroleptics (3). In spite of a careful differential diagnosis based on clinical observation and a review of the patient's history, it is likely that a small percentage of patients treated with neuroleptics will be incorrectly diagnosed as having probable tardive dyskinesia.

Patient evaluation

Following the training, all hospital patients were targeted for AIMS evaluations by teams consisting of a psychiatrist and a nurse. The examinations, which included the other movement disorders form, took ten minutes per patient. Typically, one team member administered AIMS, and both members subsequently made individual ratings of the patient. The teams produced a combined rating after any scoring discrepancies were resolved.

The team approach to AIMS ratings is not essential, but it appeared to increase scoring reliability and made the examination more instructive and enjoyable for the raters. AIMS was also incorporated into the admissions and yearly physical examination procedures at the hospital to facilitate early therapeutic intervention and provide a basis for much-needed prospective studies on the development of tardive dyskinesia.

Patient reevaluation

In the present program, hospital patients were reevaluated on AIMS by the same rater pairs roughly four months after the initial evaluation. Assessment of patients at regular intervals is useful to monitor the progress of treatment and refine the diagnosis of tardive dyskinesia. The diagnostic criteria of Schooler and Kane (12) are recommended for subsequent evaluations, particularly to distinguish between transient and persistent tardive dyskinesia.

Transient tardive dyskinesia is applicable if within three months of an evaluation the patient shows no evidence of mild to moderate tardive dyskinesia and neuroleptic dosages have remained stable or been reduced. Persistent tardive dyskinesia refers to mild to moderate symptomatology that continues over a three-month period. It should be remembered that persistent tardive dyskinesia does not mean irreversible tardive dyskinesia. Dose changes may have induced temporary fluctuations in symptomatology and the disorder may resolve later on.

Conclusion

Despite the lack of satisfactory treatment and methodology for conclusive diagnosis of tardive dyskinesia, the hospital clinician need not avoid confronting this prevalent side effect of neuroleptic medication. Mental health workers may be rapidly and reliably trained to identify subtle movement disorders using the Abnormal Involuntary Movement Scale, and taught to differentiate tardive dyskinesia from short-term neuroleptic effects and other neuromedical disorders. Subsequent patient evaluation and management may be coordinated by a part-time program administrator or by unit directors. We recommend that the AIMS evaluation be included in routine patient physical examinations to monitor the course of symptomatology over an extended period of time.

References

1. Jeste DV, Wyatt RJ: Changing epidemiology of tardive dyskinesia: an overview. American Journal of Psychiatry 138:297–309, 1981
2. Wegner JT, Kane JM: Follow-up study on the reversibility of tardive dyskinesia. American Journal of Psychiatry 139:368–369, 1982

(Continued on page 39)

Brief Reports

Identifying Subtypes
of Tardive Dyskinesia

Marion E. Wolf, M.D.
Aron D. Mosnaim, Ph.D.

Before the advent of neuroleptics, spontaneous movement disorders such as stereotypes and mannerisms were described among psychiatric patients (1). After the introduction of antipsychotic agents, a variety of drug-induced movement disorders, such as parkinsonism, akathisia, dystonias, and tardive dyskinesia, were also identified among psychiatric patients. Although tardive dyskinesia has become more prevalent, Granacher (2) has cautioned clinicians about overdiagnosing the condition, and has emphasized the importance of establishing a differential diagnosis of movement disorders.

In view of several reports on the clinical association of tardive dyskinesia and parkinsonism, the identification of concomitant drug-induced extrapyramidal side effects has also become a significant clinical issue. In addition, considerable research data support the view that there are various subtypes of tardive dyskinesia. Therefore, after conducting extended evaluations to make the diagnosis of tardive dyskinesia, clinicians must determine the type of tardive dyskinesia that a patient exhibits.

Using pharmacological probes, several investigators have identified subgroups of tardive dyskinesia (3–5). According to Casey and Denney (3), classical tardive dyskinesia is characterized by hypersensitivity of dopamine receptors and cholinergic deficits, while atypical tardive dyskinesia is characterized by dopamine deficits and excess cholinergic activity.

Gualtieri and colleagues (4) have suggested that the heterogeneous manifestations of tardive dyskinesia among children, adolescents, young adults, and older patients may reflect the existence of various subgroups of the disorder. Although tardive dyskinesia and withdrawal emergent syndrome have been described in the pediatric population, the clinical manifestations seen in children and adolescents—which include dystonic movements of the extremities, trunk, and head, and choreoathethoid and ballistic movements of the extremities—differ from those seen in the older population. The buccolingualmasticatory movements that are frequently observed in adults and particularly in elderly psychiatric patients are rarely seen in children.

Rosengarten and Friendhoff (5) demonstrated decreased dopamine receptor sensitivity in the offspring of rats treated with neuroleptics during pregnancy and observed the opposite effect in the pups when haloperidol was administered to their nursing mothers. Gualtieri and colleagues have suggested that the dopamine receptors' varied pattern of vulnerability to antipsychotic drugs administered at different developmental stages may be partly responsible for the heterogeneous clinical manifestations of tardive dyskinesia seen in subjects of different ages.

Our studies of tardive dyskinesia in adult and elderly psychiatric patients have also revealed a wide variety of clinical manifestations of the condition, supporting the view that tardive dyskinesia is a syndrome that encompasses distinct clinical entities, each with different pathogenesis, symptomatology, and response to drug therapies. Our classification of the tardive dyskinesia syndrome is based on our previous clinical findings (6–8) and also integrates previous reports by Gualtieri and colleagues (4) and Burke and colleagues (9). It identifies two main subtypes according to clinical symptomatology: choreatic tardive dyskinesia and tardive dystonia.

Based on the localization of the dyskinesia or dystonia, we can further subclassify the tardive movement disorder into orofacial, limb, and trunkal dyskinesia, and orofacial, limb, and trunkal dystonia. It should be noted, however, that, not infrequently, abnormal movements may affect more than one body area. In the following sections we shall briefly discuss the two main subtypes of tardive dyskinesia as seen in the adult population, and then characterize the subcomponents of each.

Choreatic tardive dyskinesia

This subtype of tardive dyskinesia is characterized mainly by chorea (variable, purposeless, rapid, jerky, fidgety involuntary movements); athetoses (slow, writhing, wormlike, irregular involuntary movements); and ballismus (pur-

Dr. Wolf is chief of the tardive dyskinesia program at the North Chicago Veterans Administration (VA) Medical Center, North Chicago, Illinois 60064, and associate professor of psychiatry at the University of Health Sciences/Chicago Medical School. Dr. Mosnaim is a consultant in psychiatry/research at the VA Medical Center and professor of pharmacology at the University of Health Sciences. The authors thank John M. Davis, M.D., Richard J. Wyatt, M.D., and Llewelyn Bigelow, M.D. This work was supported by grants from the VA and the Illinois Department of Mental Health.

poseless, sudden, fast, flinging involuntary movements).

Choreatic orofacial tardive dyskinesia. This is the most common variety of tardive dyskinesia in the adult population. It is characterized by abnormal movements of the face, tongue, and mouth, such as puckering and smacking of the lips, sucking and chewing movements, tongue protrusion, or choreoathethoid movements of the tongue. Since dysarthria is also a frequent symptom of this condition, it is important that clinicians note to what extent a patient's speech difficulties are due to it, or to an actual thought disorder.

Often the first early signs of tardive dyskinesia consist of abnormal buccofacialingual movements that become more frequent with advancing age. Patients report little discomfort from their movements and most are unaware of them. Pharmacologically this subtype of tardive dyskinesia seems to be the classical type (3); the dyskinesias will often become apparent upon discontinuation of neuroleptic agents and can subsequently be masked by reinstating antipsychotic drug therapy. Use of anticholinergic agents will worsen the dyskinesias or possibly convert subclinical dyskinesias into overt dyskinesias.

Choreatic limb tardive dyskinesia. Clinical manifestations of this subtype include choreoathethoid movements of the fingers and toes and the wrists and arms. Patients with this condition are also often unaware of their movement disorder and report little discomfort. It has been noted that limb dyskinesias are more commonly associated with drug-induced parkinsonism (6). In his studies of L-dopa-induced dyskinesias in patients with parkinsonism, Gerlach (10) found that the severity of the induced dyskinesias of the extremities was positively correlated with the severity of the parkinsonism in the respective extremities. He also found that limb dyskinesias were more pronounced in younger patients than were orofacial dyskinesias, which

showed an increasing rate of occurrence with age regardless of the degree of parkinsonism. Gerlach has thus suggested that while an accelerated progression of age-related changes in the oral somatotopic area of the basal ganglia is implied in the pathophysiology of oral neuroleptic-induced dyskinesias, other mechanisms are involved in the pathogenesis of limb dyskinesias.

Choreatic trunkal dyskinesia. This condition involves abnormal involuntary choreoathethoid movements affecting the neck and trunk. It is manifested by shoulder shrugging, axial hyperkinesia, and abnormal diaphragmatic movements that may cause abnormal sounds, altered voice pattern, or abnormal breathing.

Trunkal dyskinesia occurs significantly less frequently than the facial or limb dyskinesias. Its clinical manifestations are often severe, and patients will complain about their movements. Trunkal tardive dyskinesia may give the false impression of an acute pulmonary condition because of the abnormal breathing; on occasion it may result in respiratory alkalosis, physical exhaustion, and dehydration requiring intensive medical treatment.

Tardive dystonia

This second subtype of tardive dyskinesia is characterized by abnormal sustained muscular contractions that may result in slow twisting, undulant movements, or dystonic postures. Orofacial, limb, and trunkal manifestations of tardive dystonia are seen significantly less frequently in the adult population compared with the dyskinesias.

Isolated focal dystonia of the mouth, jaw, or limbs, which may result in facial disfiguration, speech problems, or abnormal positioning of the extremities, are seldom encountered. Trunkal dystonia, with or without associated face or limb dystonia, occurs slightly more frequently. Patients with trunkal dystonia may show torticollis, retrocollis, torsion

movements of the trunk, and abnormal posture and gait. These patients will definitely complain about their movement disorder. The persistent dystonia may result in osteoarthritis of the spine and intense backache.

We have also observed an association between brain damage and tardive dystonia; in terms of pathophysiology, this condition resembles atypical tardive dyskinesia (3). Thus some patients with tardive dystonia may show improvement rather than worsening of the movement disorder with the administration of anticholinergic agents. We have also postulated that deficits in phenylethlylamine may be implicated in the pathophysiology of trunkal dystonia since baclofen, B-acetic p-chlorophenylethylamine, appears to exert a selective therapeutic effect in patients with the disorder.

Conclusion

Tardive dyskinesia is a syndrome encompassing distinct clinical entities that differ in their pathogenesis, symptomatology, and response to drug treatment. Thus it is clinically of great importance not only to make the proper diagnosis of tardive dyskinesia, but to further define the subtype of tardive movement disorder.

References

1. Marsden DC, Tarsy D, Baldessarini RJ: Spontaneous and drug induced movement disorders in psychotic patients, in Psychiatric Aspects of Neurological Disease. Edited by Benson DF, Blumer D. New York, Grune & Stratton, 1975
2. Granacher RP: Differential diagnosis of tardive dyskinesia: an overview. American Journal of Psychiatry 138:1288–1297, 1981
3. Casey DE, Denney D: Pharmacological characterization of tardive dyskinesia. Psychopharmacology 54:1–8, 1977
4. Gualtieri CT, Barnhill J, McGimsey J, et al: Tardive dyskinesia and other movement disorders in children treated with psychotropic drugs. Journal of the American Academy of Child Psychiatry 19:491–510, 1980
5. Rosengarten H, Friendhoff AJ: Enduring changes in dopamine receptor cells of pups from drug administration to

(Continued on page 39)

Recognizing and Managing Akathisia

John J. Ratey, M.D.
Carl Salzman, M.D.

Akathisia is a state of motor restlessness commonly experienced as an inability to remain seated. Although akathisia was first described in 1901 and repeatedly mentioned in the psychiatric literature before the introduction of neuroleptic medication, today it is most often considered an extrapyramidal side effect of antipsychotic drugs.

Akathisia has two components, an objective state of motor restlessness and a subjective need or desire to move. The motor component is characterized by an inability to sit or stand still and by rocking, foot tapping, pacing, continual shifting from foot to foot, purposeless limb movement, coarse tremor, and even myoclonic jerks of the foot. The movements may have an extremely driven quality or may be subtle and evanescent (1). The restlessness is not localized in any part of the body and may even be voluntarily suppressed for a few moments. A similar condition is the restless legs syndrome, or the Ekbom syndrome, which produces intense subjective distress (1–3). Whether the Ekbom syndrome is a form of akathisia is not clear.

The subjective, inner state of restlessness is actually a hallmark of akathisia, although its presence is less well appreciated by clinicians. This subjective state is usually described as a feeling of restlessness, uneasiness, tension, nervousness, and jitteriness, particularly in the abdomen (4). The subjective need to move may be severe; patients describe it as feeling that they cannot sit still, are "tightened up," or are "screwed up" (1,5). A dysphoric state, resembling anxiety, is frequently a component of the inner sense of restlessness and may be difficult for patients to identify and describe. In its most severe form, the dysphoria has been associated with violent outbursts, suicide, and other strong affects such as fright, terror, anger, or rage (5–7).

Patients' descriptions of this dysphoria vary widely but attest to the extreme discomfort of akathisia: "wanting to jump out of my skin, a screaming inside" (8) or "an impending sense of implosion" (Ratey JJ, unpublished paper, 1984). For other patients there is a state of "inner driveness" that forces them to act (9). These feelings intensify the patient's focus on his or her body and the sense of being out of control, which may lead to depression, hopelessness, and the mistrust of caregivers and medications.

Because precise diagnostic criteria for akathisia do not exist, estimates of its incidence vary widely. Some authors report that 20 to 45 percent of patients taking neuroleptics have definite signs and symptoms (5,6,10–13); others believe that the incidence is much greater, that perhaps a majority of patients on neuroleptics develop akathisia (5). Akathisia is probably more common in females and in the elderly, with peak incidence in the eighth decade (14).

The profound communication difficulties of many patients receiving neuroleptics also make the incidence of akathisia difficult to determine. Patients with mental retardation, brain damage, or the cognitive deterioration and progressive withdrawal associated with chronic psychosis and hospitalization may never report any subjective distress and can give little assistance in identifying symptoms of akathisia. Some of their pacing, bizarre movements, impulsive actions, and aggressive or self-abusive behavior may be erroneously considered part of their long-standing disorder rather than a neuroleptic-induced akathisia. Thus akathisia may be particularly underdiagnosed in the chronic patient.

Akathisia's effect on the clinical state

Several reports suggest that neuroleptic-induced akathisia can worsen the clinical state of patients with schizophrenia by producing or exacerbating bizarre and impulsive behavior (5,6,11,12). Van Putten and others (12) report that 11 percent of acutely psychotic patients became more psychotic when treated with neuroleptics, with only subtle motor and subjective manifestations of akathisia present. They note that the inner restlessness of akathisia (described as "terror" by some of the patients), the bizarre body sensations, and the need to move or act can aggravate the out-of-control panic, cognitive disorganization, bodily distortions, and impulsive behavior of the psychotic state. This is particularly true for young, athletic, paranoid males, who often feel their bodies are controlled by malevolent outside forces. Additional somatic and psychic disorders induced by neuroleptics can worsen and prolong the psychotic, dysfunctional state.

Dr. Ratey is assistant director of residency training at the Massachusetts Mental Health Center, 74 Fenwood Road, Boston, Massachusetts 02115. Dr. Salzman is director of psychopharmacology at the Massachusetts Mental Health Center and associate professor of psychiatry at Harvard Medical School.

Anecdotal reports from nonpsychotic research subjects also support the view that akathisia may produce dysphoria (15–17). Kendler (15), a medical student who took a neuroleptic in a research study, poignantly expressed the intensity of akathisia's dysphoria and further remarked: "The sense of a foreign influence forcing me to move was dramatic." Other nonpsychotic subjects have reported panic attacks, agitation, reduced concentration, anxiety, and dysphoria (16). The dysphoria experienced by normal subjects has been described as a mixture of severe anxiety and tension, and a "paralysis of volition, a lack of physical and psychic energy" (18).

Clinical experience suggests there may be three groups of patients in whom akathisia often goes unrecognized and may worsen the psychosis. The first group consists of young, hostile patients, often in treatment involuntarily, who depend on physical activity to maintain a sense of self-control. They are especially likely to respond to akathisia by becoming more restless and increasingly agitated (19). In personality style these patients may resemble so-called Type A patients—those who are extraverted, self-assertive, and athletic and have a high level of physical activity, and who respond to neuroleptic drugs with increased hostility, irritability, and agitation (20,21). As these patients become more agitated, their doses of neuroleptics are commonly increased, which only exacerbates the akathisia and the agitation.

The second group consists of patients with chronic schizophrenia. They may manifest restlessness, pacing, and agitation, which can be symptoms both of schizophrenia and of akathisia. Because of cognitive impairment and reduced communication skills, they may not be able to indicate that they are experiencing the inner sense of anxiety and dysphoria associated with akathisia and thus, like the first group of patients, may be given higher doses of neuroleptics in the mistaken belief that the motor hyperactivity is part of the psychosis.

The third group of patients are those who are mentally retarded and are receiving neuroleptics for behavioral control. Like some chronic schizophrenic patients, they are unable to describe their state of inner restlessness. These patients seem particularly likely to develop acute akathisia, with agitation progressing to an "akathisia frenzy."

Diagnosis and treatment

Because of marked differences in patients' abilities to describe their inner state, the precise diagnosis of akathisia can be difficult. Akathisia usually is associated with other extrapyramidal symptoms, and the presence of parkinsonian akinesia or cogwheel rigidity may be diagnostically helpful (5,22). Braude and others (10) suggest that having the patient try to stand still for a few minutes often brings out hidden signs of motor restlessness. In patients who are able to describe inner, subjective experience, symptoms of anxiety or dysphoria should alert the clinician to akathisia.

Although extrapyramidal symptoms tend to respond to anticholinergic agents, more recent data suggest that akathisia frequently does not improve with anticholinergics (1,10,23). Benzodiazepines and amantadine have been helpful in some cases of akathisia, but the results have been inconsistent. Thus the only effective treatment is reducing the dose of the neuroleptic or discontinuing it.

In a recent study of 14 patients with neuroleptic-induced akathisia, Lipinski and others (24) reported that propranolol, in doses of 30 to 80 mg a day, was effective in diminishing akathisia symptoms in all 14 patients; nine of the 14 obtained complete remission. Ratey and others (unpublished paper, 1984) have reported successfully treating three cases of akathisia with nadolol, a long-acting peripheral beta-blocking agent, in doses of 40 to 80 mg a day. In two cases akathisia symptoms were extinguished; in the third a small dose of benzodiazepine was added to treat diminished but still bothersome symptoms of inner restlessness.

Implications for compliance

Van Putten and others (25) have suggested that akathisia may interfere with neuroleptic drug treatment. Indeed, for some patients the akathisia associated with neuroleptic treatment may be worse than any of the symptoms for which they were originally treated (26).

Since dose reduction and drug discontinuance are the only reliable treatments for akathisia, and since these steps may be countertherapeutic for the severely psychotic patient, clinicians may be faced with the difficult choice of using drugs that may actually make the patient worse or may not be taken.

Clinical experience suggests that patients who have a trusting and ongoing relationship with their treating psychiatrist may be better able to withstand drug side effects, especially akathisia. It seems likely that when the patient can acknowledge and discuss the dysphoria with the treating psychiatrist, drug compliance improves. Therefore it is important that the psychiatrist or other mental health professional discuss the symptoms of akathisia before neuroleptic treatment is begun, and continue to discuss the patient's experience during the early phases of treatment. In this manner a therapeutic alliance that incorporates joint recognition of dysphoric experience may be established. The goal is a collaboration between doctor and patient to find a dosage that combines a reduction in psychotic symptomatology with the lowest possible frequency and intensity of akathisia.

References

1. Munetz M, Cornes C: Distinguishing akathisia and tardive dyskinesia: a review of the literature. Journal of Clinical Psychopharmacology 3:343–350, 1983

2. Blom S, Ekbom KA: Comparison between akathisia developing on treatment with phenothiazine derivatives and the restless legs syndrome. Acta Medica Scandinavica 170:689–694, 1961

3. Ekbom KA: Restless legs syndrome. Neurology 10:868–873, 1960

4. Mason AS, Granacher RP: Clinical Handbook of Antipsychotic Drug Therapy. New York, Brunner/Mazel, 1980

5. Van Putten T: The many faces of akathisia. Comprehensive Psychiatry 16:43–47, 1975

6. Keckich WA: Neuroleptics: violence as a manifestation of akathisia. JAMA 240:2185, 1978

7. Shear MK, Frances A, Weiden P: Suicide associated with akathisia and depot fluphenazine treatment. Journal of Clinical Psychopharmacology 3:235–236, 1983

8. Forrest DV, Fahn S: Tardive dysphrenia and subjective akathisia (ltr). Journal of Clinical Psychiatry 40:206, 1979

9. Crane GE: Neuroleptics and their long-term side effects on the central nervous system, in Tardive Dyskinesia and Related Involuntary Movement Disorders. Edited by DeVeaugh-Geiss J. Littleton, Mass, John Wright PSG, 1982

10. Braude NVM, Barnes TR, Gore SM: Clinical characteristics of akathisia: a systematic investigation of acute psychiatric inpatient admissions. British Journal of Psychiatry 143:139–150, 1983

11. Raskin DE: Akathisia: a side effect to be remembered. American Journal of Psychiatry 129:345–347, 1972

12. Van Putten T, Mutalipassi LR, Malkin MD: Phenothiazine-induced decompensation. Archives of General Psychiatry 30:102–105, 1974

13. Ayd FJ: A survey of extrapyramidal drug-induced reactions. JAMA 175:1054–1060, 1961

14. Salzman C, Shader RI, Pearlman M: Psychopharmacology and the elderly, in Psychotropic Drug Side Effects. Edited by Shader RI, DiMascio A. Baltimore, Williams & Wilkins, 1970

15. Kendler KS: A medical student's experience with akathisia. American Journal of Psychiatry 133:454–455, 1976

16. Anderson BG, Reker D, Cooper T: Prolonged adverse effects of haloperidol in normal subjects. New England Journal of Medicine 305:643–644, 1981

17. Van Putten T, May PRA, Marder SR, et al: Subjective response to antipsychotic drugs. Archives of General Psychiatry 38:187–190, 1981

18. Belmaker R, Wald D: Haloperidol in normals (ltr). British Journal of Psychiatry 131:222–223, 1977

19. Sarwer-Foner G: Recognition and management of drug-induced extrapyramidal reactions and "paradoxical" behavioral reactions in psychiatry. Canadian Medical Association Journal 83:312–318, 1960

20. Heninger G, DiMascio A, Klerman GL: Personality factors in variability of response to phenothiazines. American Journal of Psychiatry 122:1091–1094, 1965

21. DiMascio A, Bernardo DL, Greenblatt DJ, et al: A controlled trial of amantadine in drug-induced extrapyramidal disorders. Archives of General Psychiatry 33:599–602, 1976

22. Maltbie AA, Cavenar JO Jr: Akathisia diagnosis: an objective test. Psychosomatics 18:36–39, 1977

23. Neurological syndromes associated with antipsychotic drug use: a special report. Archives of General Psychiatry 28:463–467, 1973

24. Lipinski JF, Zubenko GS, Cohen BM, et al: Propranolol in the treatment of neuroleptic-induced akathisia. American Journal of Psychiatry 141:412–415, 1964

25. Van Putten T, May PRA, Marder SR: Response to antipsychotic medication: the doctor's and the consumer's view. American Journal of Psychiatry 141:16–19, 1984

26. Kalinowsky LB: Appraisal of the "tranquilizers" and their influence on other somatic treatments in psychiatry. American Journal of Psychiatry 115:294–300, 1958

A Clinical Guide for Diagnosing and Managing Patients With Drug-Induced Dysphagia

Peter Weiden, M.D.
Maura Harrigan, M.S., R.D.

Both Parkinson's disease and tardive dyskinesia have been shown to cause a wide range of eating and swallowing disturbances that can result in life-threatening complications, such as sudden choking, aspiration, and malnutrition (1,2). Dysphagia, or difficulty swallowing, is a most reliable symptom and should not be dismissed as an emotional disturbance (3). Psychotropic medications are etiologically implicated in the swallowing disorders of patients with Parkinson's disease and tardive dyskinesia by a variety of pathophysiologic factors.

First, dysphagia is present in up to 50 percent of patients with Parkinson's disease, and complications from dysphagia are a frequent cause of death among these patients. The anatomic basis of swallowing dysfunction is demonstrated radiographically in the proximal pharyngeal and esophageal musculature (2). It is thought that these areas are predominantly under central dopaminergic control and treatable with antiparkinsonian agents. By blocking dopaminergic transmission, neuroleptic

Dr. Weiden is a clinical instructor in psychiatry at the Payne Whitney Psychiatric Clinic in New York City and Ms. Harrigan is assistant director of nutrition services at St. Vincent's Hospital and Medical Center in New York City. Address correspondence to Dr. Weiden at the Department of Psychiatry, New York Hospital–Cornell Medical Center, 525 East 68th Street, New York, New York 10021.

drugs may cause a dysphagia clinically identical to that caused by Parkinson's disease alone.

Second, choreiform movement disorders that are characteristic of tardive dyskinesia are thought to arise from postsynaptic dopaminergic supersensitivity (4). Both lingual and upper esophageal hyperkinesias with obvious potential for disruption of normal swallowing mechanisms have been observed in patients with tardive dyskinesia (5). Additionally, the anticholinergic agents that are frequently used in conjunction with neuroleptics may impair the gag reflex and contribute to dysphagia and choking deaths (6).

Despite the potential seriousness of dysphagia, we do not know of a clinical guide for diagnosing and managing patients with drug-induced swallowing disorders. But as the case report below illustrates, simple and practical diagnostic and therapeutic maneuvers are available for use with these patients. Following the case report, we will suggest guidelines for evaluating and treating patients with drug-induced swallowing disorders.

Case report

Ms. A is a 71-year-old woman with multiple hospitalizations for exacerbations of chronic paranoid schizophrenia. During her last psychotic episode and subsequent hospitalization, in 1980, mild orobuccal tardive dyskinesia was noted. Since then she has been receiving fluphenazine 15 mg a day and benztropine 2 mg a day as an outpatient. Attempts were made to taper her fluphenazine, but after a few months her psychotic symptoms recurred.

In 1983, however, Ms. A's movement disorder progressed, and she developed severe neck and truncal dystonias. At the same time she began having difficulty swallowing solid foods and had to cut her food into smaller pieces. She showed no weight loss and did not have a history of dysphagia or other gastrointestinal symptoms. Her past medical history was unremarkable, and her physical examination, including the gag reflex, was normal except for symptoms of tardive dyskinesia and drug-induced parkinsonism.

A second attempt to taper Ms. A's neuroleptic medication resulted in rapid worsening of her dyskinetic symptoms; she had acute dyspnea and was unable to swallow any solid food. Her psychiatric status was unchanged except for increased anxiety. Increasing the fluphenazine quickly reversed this dramatic presentation and resolved her respiratory and pharyngeal symptoms.

Nevertheless, Ms. A's dysphagia progressed over the following year, and her weight went from her baseline of 128 pounds to 98 pounds—23 percent below ideal body weight. She reported difficulty swallowing particulate foods that flake or crumble. Her appetite and ability to swallow liquids remained intact, and her gag reflex was preserved. She was placed on a nutritionally complete liquid supplement (1,440 calories per day) and showed a dramatic response, going back to 114 pounds in five weeks. Based on this response we felt no further medical workup was necessary.

Discussion

Swallowing is divided into the oral, pharyngeal, and esophageal stages, each of which has a separate function (3). In the oral stage the bolus is formed and positioned over the tongue, which then initiates the swallowing reflex. During the pharyngeal phase the bolus is prevented from entering the larynx by finely coordinated contractions of tongue, posterior pharyngeal, and epiglottal musculature. The esophageal stage marks the beginning of peristaltic movements. This complex mechanism can be disturbed by either hypokinetic movements of parkinsonism or hyperkinetic choreas of tardive dyskinesia. For example, lingual tardive dyskinesia interferes with the normal mouth control of food during bolus formation.

The type and degree of dysphagia must be assessed in every patient suspected of drug-induced dysphagia. Table 1 provides a clinical guide to evaluation and treatment by showing the symptoms of dysphagia found in each of the swallowing phases and the recommended clinical action for each symptom. The two most important factors to assess are the presence of a gag reflex and mouth control to form an adequate bolus (7). Absence of a gag reflex indicates a high risk of aspiration and contraindicates liquid supplementation.

When checking the gag reflex, it is helpful to observe the patient swallowing a liquid. It is normal for the head to tilt slightly forward during drinking; any deviation from this position suggests an impaired gag reflex. The clinician should ask about and look for coughing that may follow ingestion of particulate foods, which implies poor epiglottal coordination (8).

The goal of nutritional management of patients with drug-induced swallowing disorders is to provide adequate calories and protein to prevent malnutrition in a way that best avoids aspiration. Nutritional consultation with a registered dietitian is advised so that a feeding program based on the type and degree of swallowing impairment is designed (9). If the gag reflex is impaired, the patient may have to avoid liquids and particulate foods such as hamburger, hard rolls, fried foods, and crisp salads. If bolus formation is impaired, soft and cohesive foods that require little or no chewing, such as pudding, custard, firm gelatin, oatmeal, pureed food, fruit nectars, and thick soups, are indicated.

When caloric supplementation is

Table 1
Clinical guide for evaluating neuroleptic-induced dysphagia

Swallowing stage and symptoms of dysphagia	Recommendation
Oral	
Inadequate saliva Bolus inadequately lubricated	Examine oral cavity for hyperkinetic movements, dryness of mucous membranes, dentition, and other lesions
Difficulty chewing Bolus inadequately formed	Evaluate neuroleptic and anticholinergic status
Lip smacking Premature initiation of swallowing reflex	Provide moist and cohesive foods in small amounts
Tongue vermiform movement, thrusting, or both Bolus inadequately formed	
Pharyngeal	
Coughing Aspiration risk	Check gag reflex
Regurgitation Aspiration risk	Look for palatal and uvular dyskinesias
Choking Aspiration risk	Evaluate neuroleptic and anticholinergic status Ask for history of pneumonia or choking Evaluate tolerance of liquids and particulate foods by taking history and by observing patient swallowing
Esophageal	
Halitosis	Ask for history of symptoms
Nocturnal asthma	Evaluate neuroleptic and anticholinergic status
Nocturnal vomiting Aspiration risk Status of food in esophagus	

needed, the patient can purchase nutritionally complete, over-the-counter liquids that supply protein, fat, and carbohydrate as well as vitamins and minerals. Nutritional puddings can be substituted for liquids when the gag reflex is impaired. Meals may have to be supervised and the patient's weight and other nutritional parameters followed.

It is important to obtain the patient's medication history to determine whether the dysphagia is caused by tardive dyskinesia or drug-induced parkinsonism. The correct diagnosis has important treatment implications. Although the goal of pharmacologic therapy of a drug-induced dysphagia is removal of the precipitating agent, typically dysphagia from tardive

dyskinesia worsens when the neuroleptic dosage is lowered. The opposite is true for drug-induced parkinsonism. The absence of an expected response to a change in neuroleptics warrants medical consultation to rule out other etiologies of the dysphagia.

Ms. A's case demonstrates some of the problems involved in clinical assessment. Her psychiatric status compromised her ability to report her swallowing difficulties and consequently they came to our attention late. Once she was diagnosed as dysphagic, we had to determine whether the dysphagia was caused by parkinsonism, tardive dyskinesia, anticholinergics, or an unrelated medical illness. It was only the rapid progression of dysphagia following neuroleptic withdrawal that established that the dysphagia was due to tardive dyskinesia.

We recommend routinely asking patients with severe tardive dyskinesia or parkinsonism about difficulty swallowing and routinely following their weights. We also recommend careful oral and pharyngeal examination, especially of the gag reflex, for all psychiatric patients maintained on neuroleptics since asphyxia deaths may also occur in asymptomatic patients with no prior history of dysphagia (10).

References

1. Moss HB, Green A: Neuroleptic-associated dysphagia confirmed by esophageal manometry. American Journal of Psychiatry 139:515–516, 1982
2. Lieberman AN, Horowitz L, Redmond P, et al: Dysphagia in Parkinson's disease. American Journal of Gastroenterology 74:157–160, 1980
3. Isselbacher KJ, Adams RD, Braunwald E, et al (eds): Harrison's Principles of Internal Medicine, 9th ed. New York, McGraw Hill, 1980
4. Tarsy D, Baldessarini RF: The pathophysiologic basis of tardive dyskinesia. Biological Psychiatry 12:431–450, 1977
5. Massengill R, Nashold B: A swallowing disorder denoted in tardive dyskinesia patients. Acta Otolaryngologica 68:457–458, 1969
6. Craig TJ, Richardson MA: Swallowing, tardive dyskinesia, and anticholinergics (ltr). American Journal of Psychiatry 139:1083, 1982
7. Hargrove R: Feeding the severely dysphagic patient. Journal of Neurosurgical Nursing 12:102–107, 1980
8. Buckley JE, Addicks CC, Maniglia J: Feeding patients with dysphagia. Nursing Forum 15:69–85, 1976
9. Logeman J: Evaluation and Treatment of Dysphagia. San Diego, College Hill Press, 1983
10. Craig TJ: Medication use and deaths attributed to asphyxia among psychiatric patients. American Journal of Psychiatry 137:1366–1373, 1980

Brief Reports

(Continued from page 33)

pregnant and nursing rats. Science 203:1133–1135, 1979
6. Wolf ME, Chevesich J, Lehrer E, et al: The clinical association of tardive dyskinesia and drug induced parkinsonism. Biological Psychiatry 18:1181–1188, 1983
7. Wolf ME, Chevesich J, Mosnaim AD: Trunkal tardive dyskinesia. Neurology 33(Suppl 2):198, 1983
8. Wolf ME, Keener S, Mathis P, et al: Phenylethylamine-like properties of baclofen. Neuropsychobiology 9:219–222, 1983
9. Burke RE, Fahn S, Jankovic J, et al: Tardive dystonia: late onset and persistent dystonia caused by antipsychotic drugs. Neurology 32:1335–1346, 1982
10. Gerlach J: The relationship between parkinsonism and tardive dyskinesia. American Journal of Psychiatry 134:781–784, 1977

Law & Psychiatry

(Continued from page 29)

5. Faigenbaum v Oakland Medical Center, Association of Trial Lawyers of America Law Reporter 25:473, 1982
6. Gutheil TG, Appelbaum PS: "Mind control," "synthetic sanity," "artificial competence," and genuine confusion: legally relevant effects of antipsychotic medication. Hofstra Law Review 12:77–120, 1983
7. Wettstein RM: Tardive dyskinesia and malpractice. Behavioral Sciences and the Law 1:85–107, 1983
8. Charles SC, Wilbert JR, Kennedy EC: Physicians' self-reports of reactions to malpractice litigation. American Journal of Psychiatry 141:563–565, 1984
9. Kalachnik JE, Larum JG, Swanson A: Brief report: a tardive dyskinesia monitoring policy for applied facilities. Psychopharmacology Bulletin 19:277–282, 1983
10. Press I: The predisposition to file claims: the patient's perspective. Law, Medicine, and Health Care 12:53–62, 1984

Psychopharmacology

(Continued from page 31)

3. Kane JM, Smith JM: Tardive dyskinesia: prevalence and risk factors. Archives of General Psychiatry 39:473–481, 1982
4. DeVeaugh-Geiss J: Epidemiology of tardive dyskinesia: I, in Tardive Dyskinesia and Related Involuntary Movement Disorders. Edited by DeVeaugh-Geiss J. Boston, John Wright, 1982
5. Jeste DV, Wyatt RJ: In search of treatment for tardive dyskinesia: review of the literature. Schizophrenia Bulletin 5:251–293, 1979
6. Smith JM, Baldessarini RJ: Changes in prevalence, severity, and recovery in tardive dyskinesia with age. Archives of General Psychiatry 37:1368–1373, 1980
7. Casey DE, Toenniessen L: Tardive dyskinesia: what is the natural history? International Drug Therapy Newsletter 18:13–16, 1983
8. Jeste DV, Wyatt RJ: Therapeutic strategies against tardive dyskinesia. Archives of General Psychiatry 39:803–816, 1982
9. Guy W: ECDEU Assessment Manual for Psychopharmacology. Washington, DC, US Department of Health, Education, and Welfare, 1976
10. Smith JM, Kucharski LT, Oswald WT, et al: A systematic investigation of tardive dyskinesia in inpatients. American Journal of Psychiatry 136:918–922, 1979
11. Chien C-P, Jung K, Ross-Townsend A, et al: The measurement of persistent dyskinesia by piezoelectric recording and clinical rating scales. Psychopharmacology Bulletin 13:34–36, 1977
12. Schooler NR, Kane JM: Research diagnosis for tardive dyskinesia. Archives of General Psychiatry 39:486–487, 1982
13. Granacher RP: Differential diagnosis of tardive dyskinesia: an overview. American Journal of Psychiatry 138:1288–1297, 1981
14. American Psychiatric Association: Tardive dyskinesia: summary of a task force report. American Journal of Psychiatry 137:1163–1171, 1980
15. Smith JM, Kucharski LT, Eblin C, et al: An assessment of tardive dyskinesia in schizophrenic outpatients. Psychopharmacology 64:99–104, 1979
16. Smith JM, Oswald WT, Kucharski LT, et al: Tardive dyskinesia: age and sex differences in hospitalized schizophrenics. Psychopharmacology 58:207–211, 1978
17. Rosen AM, Mukherjee S, Olarte S, et al: Perception of tardive dyskinesia in outpatients receiving maintenance neuroleptics. American Journal of Psychiatry 139:372–373, 1982
18. Jus A, Jus K, Fontaine P: Long-term treatment of tardive dyskinesia. Journal of Clinical Psychiatry 40:72–77, 1979
19. Seeman, MV: Tardive dyskinesia: two-year recovery. Comprehensive Psychiatry 22:189–192, 1981

APA Statement on Tardive Dyskinesia

Tardive dyskinesia (TD) is a syndrome of choreoathetoid and/or other involuntary movements that may affect mouth, lips, tongue, arms, legs, or trunk; tardive dyskinesia is associated with the long-term (usually greater than six months) use of neuroleptics.

The proportion of patients developing abnormal involuntary movements is believed to increase with increasing length of treatment or total exposure to neuroleptics. The syndrome can develop after relatively brief (three to six months) treatment periods at low dosages. However, it is impossible at present to identify which patients are at risk.

In cross-sectional studies, the majority of cases are judged to be mild (i.e., not obvious to the untrained observer or subjectively troublesome to the patient).

Identification and diagnosis are complicated by the fact that neuroleptic drugs may mask TD symptoms. Drug discontinuation or dosage reduction may reveal previously masked symptoms.

Although there are few long-term follow-up studies, the condition does not appear to be generally progressive. The prevalence of tardive dyskinesia does increase with age.

The course of the condition is difficult to predict in individual patients. Though some cases will have symptoms resolved, a proportion of patients will show persistent dyskinesias even after drug discontinuation.

There is no established treatment for tardive dyskinesia.

Recommendations for the use of neuroleptics

Long-term use of neuroleptics is primarily indicated in schizophrenia, paranoia, childhood psychoses, and certain neuropsychiatric disorders such as Gilles de La Tourette's syndrome and Huntington's disease. Short-term administration (less than six months) is justifiable in many cases of acute psychotic episode, severe mania or agitated depression, and certain organic mental disorders. Rarely, patients with other conditions who have not responded to alternative treatments may benefit from the use of neuroleptics.

All patients receiving long-term treatment require periodic evaluation and documentation of continued need and benefit.

The benefits and risks of long-term treatment should be discussed with patients and families and their informed consent to treatment documented.

Patients should be routinely examined for signs of tardive dyskinesia.

Neuroleptic drugs should be administered at the lowest effective dosage. Attempts at dosage reduction and in some cases (depending upon clinical state, past history, etc.) drug discontinuation should be considered.

Concerned about patients' risk of developing tardive dyskinesia with long-term use of neuroleptic drugs, in 1985 the American Psychiatric Association's Task Force on Tardive Dyskinesia issued this statement summarizing information about the movement disorder and containing recommendations for the use of neuroleptics.